Federico Alvarez Igarzábal, Chad Comeau, Emmanuel Guardiola, Carmen Johann, Katharina Tillmanns (eds.)
Video Games and Mental Health



**Studies of Digital Media Culture** | 18

The series is edited by Gundolf S. Freyermuth and Lisa Gotto.

**Federico Alvarez Igarzábal** is Professor of Digital Media & Game Studies at the University of Fine Arts Essen (HBK Essen). His research straddles the humanities and the natural sciences, combining theoretical and experimental approaches to examine the temporal aesthetics of video games and the mental state of play.
**Chad Comeau** is a researcher at the Cologne Game Lab (TH Köln, Germany), creative director at Reframe Games, and leads interactive cultural projects through his company Fring Frang Games. Bringing over a decade of professional experience in game design, project management and languages, Chad tackles various societal and cultural issues in his work.
**Emmanuel Guardiola** is a veteran of the video game industry with more than 30 major titles published for publishers such as Ubisoft and independent studios. He holds a PhD in computer science and is professor at the Cologne Game Lab, TH Köln (Cologne University of Applied Sciences, Germany). In the field of game design research, he is interested in models, processes, and characteristics of the gameplay experience, and how we can apply these findings to education, health, psychology, or humanitarian causes.
**Carmen Johann** is a game designer, UX designer, and researcher in the field of digital learning, specializing in user-centered learning systems, serious games, and interactive educational media.
**Katharina Tillmanns** is a researcher, designer, and curator working at the intersection of games, psychology, and embodied media. She is a lecturer at the Cologne Game Lab, TH Köln, and a doctoral candidate at University of Cologne where her research explores Mixed Reality design with a focus on affect, emotional engagement, and user well-being. Across her projects and publications, Tillmanns advances the idea of games as both artistic and epistemic media, with the potential to support psychological insight, foster empathy, and open new pathways for education and well-being.

Federico Alvarez Igarzábal, Chad Comeau, Emmanuel Guardiola,
Carmen Johann, Katharina Tillmanns (eds.)

# Video Games and Mental Health

Perspectives of Psychology and Game Design

[transcript]

This project was funded by the German Federal Ministry of Education and Research (FKZ:13FH037SA7).

**Bibliographic information published by the Deutsche Nationalbibliothek**
The Deutsche Nationalbibliothek lists this publication in the Deutsche Nationalbibliografie; detailed bibliographic data are available online at https://dnb.dnb.de



transcript Verlag | Hermannstraße 26 | D-33602 Bielefeld | live@transcript-verlag.de

Cover design: Maria Arndt
Cover illustration: © Carmen Johann
Printing: Druckhaus Bechstein GmbH, Wetzlar
https://doi.org/10.14361/9783839468562
Print-ISBN: 978-3-8376-6856-8 | PDF-ISBN: 978-3-8394-6856-2
ISSN of series: 2702-8240 | eISSN of series: 2702-8259

Printed on permanent acid-free text paper.

# Contents

## Design Perspectives



## Appendix

# Video Games and Mental Health
## Introduction

*Federico Alvarez Igarzábal, Chad Comeau, Emmanuel Guardiola, Carmen Johann and Katharina Tillmanns*

In recent years, mental health and well-being have emerged as key concerns in the global games industry. Academic interest in this topic has also increased, addressing open questions as to how video games affect our mental health, both positively and negatively (Ballou et al., 2025). While collaborations between the industry and academia are still rare, they are crucial to develop a full understanding of the impact that video games are having on players (Johannes et al., 2021). The impact of video games has been historically understood to be negative, with claims of games causing violence or addiction—the former has been fully debunked (Markey & Ferguson, 2017), while the second remains an open question.[1] More recent research has shown, contrary to popular belief, that video games can improve our mental health (Kowal et al., 2021; Kowert et al., 2021).

The COVID-19 pandemic made questions concerning the impact of video games in our mental well-being even more urgent, with many seeking support in entertainment media and online communities (Dunlap, 2022). As people around the world faced isolation, uncertainty, and stress, they turned to games for connection, safety, and emotional relief. In this context, the World Health Organization (WHO) teamed up with gaming industry leaders to launch the campaign #PlayApartTogether (2020) on social media. This campaign promoted the use of WHO's health guidelines while encouraging people to stay connected through games during periods where social distancing was required. In a survey by DiFrancisco-Donoghue and colleagues (2023), 74.6% of participants reported playing more video games during the beginning of the pandemic. A further study by Barr & Copeland-Stewart (2022) showed that the numbers of people gaming during the pandemic increased,

1 Some scholars contend that games are addictive and others that the evidence is still insufficient to reach a conclusion (see Zastrow, 2017). Scholars in the latter group have also expressed concerns that the inclusion of the "Gaming Disorder" diagnosis in the WHO's International Classification of Diseases-11 is premature, potentially doing more harm than good (Van Rooij et al., 2018).

and that people played more on average. The study also showed that gaming during the pandemic had overall positive effects on mental health. This has led to an increase in the demand for games that address mental health (Kowal et al., 2021), which can be addressed both by *applied games* and *entertainment games*.

Applied games are created with a specific purpose beyond having fun—such as education, training, or therapy. In the context of psychology, applied games are often informed by knowledge from clinical research, digital health tools, therapy methods, and self-help practices. These games aim to provide accessible and innovative ways for users to understand and manage their mental health. Some are developed as tools to diagnose psychological conditions, help treat mental illnesses, or train specific emotional skills. Others are used by researchers and clinicians to study behavior, assess personality traits, or simulate social and emotional responses. These games combine psychology and technology to create useful tools for health professionals and individuals alike. Some notable examples in this category are PROJECT SPARX (see Merry et al., 2012), ENDEAVOR XR (Kollins et al., 2020, 2021), and the work of Isabela Granic and coworkers at the GEMH (Games for Emotional and Mental Health) Lab (see for instance Tsui et al., 2021). And research projects like VIRTUALTIMES (2019–2023) are producing valuable insights into how to develop video games and virtual environments for therapeutic purposes.[2]

The entertainment games industry, while still being primarily in the business of creating tools for escapism, is also showing an increased concern with mental health. Many *indie* game developers today are creating personal and emotionally rich experiences that reflect their own stories or the stories of people close to them. Following the tradition of *games d'auteur*, the vision and voice of a single creator or a small group of creators are at the center of these titles. Such games often include characters who experience depression, anxiety, or trauma, helping players explore complex emotions and situations from a personal point of view. By engaging with these experiences, players can also learn more about mental health, develop empathy, and feel part of a shared conversation. These games may not aim to "fix" problems, but they offer meaningful stories that can reduce stigma and help players feel seen and understood. A video game in this vein that garnered much attention in the press and academia is HELLBLADE: SENUA'S SACRIFICE (Ninja Theory, 2017), which features a main character who suffers from psychosis. The development team sought counsel from neuroscientists to create an accurate representation of its phenomenology (Brierley, 2021). Sébastien Genvo's Expressive Game Lab specializes in delivering this sort of experience. This volume includes a chapter authored by Genvo on LIE IN MY HEART (Expressive Gamestudio 2019), a game through which the author expressed and processed his grief after his wife, who suffered from

2 Full disclosure: Federico Alvarez Igarzábal, co-editor of this volume, was involved in the VIRTUALTIMES project.

bipolar disorder, took her own life. Another title discussed in this anthology's pages is DURU (Twisted Ramble Games UG, 2023; see Kerstin Schütt's chapter COLORFUL DEPRESSION), which tells a personal story of battling with depression. In the realm of acade-mia, the project UNDERSTANDING VIDEO GAME PLAY AND MENTAL HEALTH (2023–2025) stands out as a successful cooperation between scholars and the industry that produced insightful research on the effects of commercial video games on player well-being.

The volume in your hands examines current trends and future directions at the intersection of game design and mental health. It is divided into three parts: *Positive Impact*, *Representation*, and *Designer Perspectives*.

## Positive impact

The first section of the book looks at the positive effects that video games can have on mental health and well-being. It shows how games can help improve players' emotions, encourage personal growth, and promote healthy behaviors. Nicholas D. Bowman, Jordan King, Tim Wulf, and Sarah Hodge explore the positive impact of nostalgia in video gaming. Maude Bonenfant, Élisa Vial, and Clara Lhotellier analyze the social phenomenon of peer support in online gaming communities. Marco Rüth offers an insightful overview of the research on how video games and gamified apps can promote healthy and pro-environmental behavior. And Richy Srirachanikorn examines how a game like HIKIKOMORI LIFE (Micro Team Games, 2022) can help players understand social isolation.

## Representation

The second section focuses on how video games represent different psychological and social issues. It examines how games handle serious topics like loss, addiction, and mental illness, and how these portrayals can help players understand and empathize with those going through such situations. Kelli Dunlap and Christopher Leech offer a descriptive analysis of different ways in which video games can represent the experience of grief and offer important insights into this psychological state produced by significant loss (especially of a loved one). Danielle Kelly and Bethany Thomas examine the representation of female protagonists in video games through the lens of stereotype theory. Tero Kerttula analyzes the representation of alcoholism in PSYCHONAUTS 2. And Stefan Simond looks into the use of sanity as a resource in horror video games and the representations of madness thar ensue when this resource depletes.

## Design perspectives

The third section presents game-design approaches to dealing with mental health themes. It explores how designers create games that talk about serious topics like depression, suicide, and resilience. It also discusses how games can be used to raise awareness and help players better understand mental health. By sharing the views of game creators who intentionally include mental health topics in their work, this section offers a sample of texts that illustrate the growing role that psychopathology plays in the game industry, highlighting the responsibility that designers have to approach these themes thoughtfully and compassionately. Sébastien Genvo discusses the development of LIE IN MY HEART, a deeply personal game about suicide and grief. Kerstin Schütt offers insights into the design of DURU – ABOUT MOLE RATS AND DEPRESSION and offers a step-by-step guide on how to create games that deal with serious topics. And Samantha Accettulli examines how DISCO ELYSIUM (ZA/UM, 2019) deals with dissociative disorder and can help players cope with their own mental health struggles. Through these insights, the section shows how games can be a tool for personal reflection and emotional growth.

By bringing together an array of international perspectives from different disciplines, VIDEO GAMES AND MENTAL HEALTH shows how the leading entertainment medium of our time is used in innovative ways to engage with personal and social issues that impact psychological well-being. It includes a wide range of case studies, theoretical discussions, empirical research, game design approaches, and practical applications. By looking at both applied and entertainment games, its chapters offer a wide-ranging perspective on how games can support mental health and offer psychological insights. Contributions stem from academic research, industry projects, and interdisciplinary collaborations between these two worlds. The ultimate goal of this volume is to connect ideas and experiences across fields, and to help readers understand how games can be used to explore the human mind, promote emotional well-being, and support mental health in creative and meaningful ways.

## Acknowledgements

First and foremost, we extend our heartfelt thanks to the contributors to this volume for their dedication. Their thoughtful and insightful articles shape this multidisciplinary anthology. We thank the German Federal Ministry of Education and Research (BMBF) for its financial support of this publication and the research project SOLVE, within the framework of the funding line FH-Sozial 2017. Our sincere gratitude goes Laura Frings, CGL's Research Coordinator, for her support securing this funding. We thank Anna-Lena Richter for her collaboration on the book's layouting. We are grateful to the Cologne Game Lab and its Clash of Realities conference, which provided the forum that ultimately made this publication possible. We deeply appreciate Gundolf S. Freyermuth and Lisa Gotto for including our work in the Studies of Digital Media Culture series at transcript. Finally, we would like to thank transcript Publishing and in particular our editor, Annika Linnemann, for the support throughout the publication process.

## References

#PlayApartTogether (2020, March 29). *Games Industry Unites to Promote World Health Organization Messages Against COVID-19; Launch #PlayApartTogether Campaign.* Medium. https://medium.com/@playaparttogether/games-industry-unites-to-promote-world-health-organization-messages-against-covid-19-launch-bfc6fc611641

Ballou, N., Hakman, T., Vuorre, M., Magnusson, K., & Przybylski, A. K. (2025). How do video games affect mental health? A narrative review of 13 proposed mechanisms. *Technology, Mind, and Behavior*, 6(2). https://doi.org/10.1037/tmb0000152

Barr, M., & Copeland-Stewart, A. (2022). Playing Video Games During the COVID-19 Pandemic and Effects on Players' Well-Being. *Games and Culture*, 17(1), 122–139. https://doi.org/10.1177/15554120211017036

Brierley, C. (2021, September 30). *The Pict warrior fighting her inner demons.* University of Cambridge. https://www.cam.ac.uk/stories/hellblade-innerdemons

DiFrancisco-Donoghue, J., De Las Heras, B., Li, O., Middleton, J., & Jung, M.-K. (2023). Gaming in Pandemic Times: An International Survey Assessing the Effects of COVID-19 Lockdowns on Young Video Gamers' Health. *International Journal of Environmental Research and Public Health*, 20(19), 6855. https://doi.org/10.3390/ijerph20196855

Dunlap, K. (2022). Mental Health of Twitch Streamers During COVID-19. In J. Aguilar Rodríguez, F. Alvarez Igarzábal, M. S. Debus, C. L. Maughan, S.-J. Song, M. Vozaru, & F. Zimmermann (Hrsg.), *Mental Health | Atmospheres | Video Games. New Directions in Game Research II* (1. Aufl., S. 103–116). transcript Verlag. https://doi.org/10.14361/9783839462645-010

Johannes, N., Vuorre, M., & Przybylski, A. K. (2021). Video game play is positively correlated with well-being. *Royal Society Open Science*, 8(2). https://doi.org/10.1098/rsos.202049

Kollins, S. H., Childress, A., Heusser, A. C., & Lutz, J. (2021). Effectiveness of a digital therapeutic as adjunct to treatment with medication in pediatric ADHD. *Npj Digital Medicine*, 4(1). https://doi.org/10.1038/s41746-021-00429-0

Kollins, S. H., DeLoss, D. J., Cañadas, E., Lutz, J., Findling, R. L., Keefe, R. S. E., Epstein, J. N., Cutler, A. J., & Faraone, S. V. (2020). A novel digital intervention for actively reducing severity of paediatric ADHD (STARS-ADHD): A randomised controlled trial. *The Lancet Digital Health*, 2(4), e168–e178. https://doi.org/10.1016/s2589-7500(20)30017-0

Kowal, M., Conroy, E., Ramsbottom, N., Smithies, T., Toth, A., & Campbell, M. (2021). Gaming Your Mental Health: A Narrative Review on Mitigating Symptoms of Depression and Anxiety Using Commercial Video Games. *JMIR Serious Games*, 9(2), e26575. https://doi.org/10.2196/26575

Kowert, R., Ferguson, C. J., Fletcher, P. C., & Rusch, D. (2021). Editorial: Digital Games and Mental Health. *Frontiers in Psychology*, 12. https://doi.org/10.3389/fpsyg.2021.713107

Markey, P. M., & Ferguson, C. J. (2017). *Moral combat: Why the war on violent video games is wrong*. BenBella Books, Inc.

Merry, S. N., Stasiak, K., Shepherd, M., Frampton, C., Fleming, T., & Lucassen, M. F. G. (2012). The effectiveness of SPARX, a computerised self help intervention for adolescents seeking help for depression: Randomised controlled non-inferiority trial. *BMJ*, *344*(apr18 3), e2598–e2598. https://doi.org/10.1136/bmj.e2598

Micro Team Games. (2022). HIKIKOMORI LIFE. [PC]. Steam.

Ninja Theory (2019). HELLBLADE: SENUA'S SACRIFICE. Ninja Theory.

Tsui, T. Y. L., DeFrance, K., Khalid-Khan, S., Granic, I., & Hollenstein, T. (2021). Reductions of Anxiety Symptoms, State Anxiety, and Anxious Arousal in Youth Playing the Videogame MindLight Compared to Online Cognitive Behavioral Therapy. *Games for Health Journal*. https://doi.org/10.1089/g4h.2020.0083

Twisted Ramble Games UG (2023). DURU – ABOUT MOLE RATS AND DEPRESSION. Twisted Ramble Games UG.

Understanding Video Game Play and Mental Health (2023–2025). Oxford Internet Institute. https://www.oii.ox.ac.uk/research/projects/understanding-videogame-play-and-mental-health/

VIRTUALTIMES. Exploring and Modifying the Sense of Time in Virtual Environments (2019–2023). CORDIS. https://cordis.europa.eu/project/id/824128

Van Rooij, A. J., Ferguson, C. J., Colder Carras, M., Kardefelt-Winther, D., Shi, J., Aarseth, E., Bean, A. M., Bergmark, K. H., Brus, A., Coulson, M., Deleuze, J., Dullur, P., Dunkels, E., Edman, J., Elson, M., Etchells, P. J., Fiskaali, A., Granic, I., Jansz, J., … Przybylski, A. K. (2018). A weak scientific basis for gaming disorder: Let us err on the side of caution. *Journal of Behavioral Addictions*, 7(1), 1–9. https://doi.org/10.1556/2006.7.2018.19

Zastrow, M. (2017). Is video game addiction really an addiction? *Proceedings of the National Academy of Sciences*, *114*(17), 4268–4272. https://doi.org/10.1073/pnas.1705077114

ZA/UM (2021). DISCO ELYSIUM: THE FINAL CUT. ZA/UM.

# Positive Impact

# "Take Eight Bits and Call Me in the Morning"

## Video Games, Well-Being, and the Psychology of Nostalgia

*Nicholas D. Bowman, Tim Wulf, Jordan King and Sarah Hodge*

For nearly 60 years, video games have arrested the attention of players, inviting us to interact and interface with on-screen content. More than just short-term entertainment experiences, video games are part of a broader cultural milieu—they are the most profitable media entertainment sector (global revenues nearly $400 billion USD in 2023) with more than 3.5 billion players globally (Clement, 2023). Similar to other entertainment media, some video game intellectual properties have transcended generations and, in many cases, grown beyond the medium itself: common cultural touchstones include SUPER MARIO BROS. and SONIC THE HEDGEHOG, along with seemingly endless subcultures of devoted fans of specific games and gaming properties (Jenkins, 2006). Unique from other entertainment media, video games present as "digital time machines" that allow players to directly revisit personally relevant and highly familiar worlds from the past in which those worlds remain unchanged (Robinson & Bowman, 2021; Wulf et al., 2018).

Among the many outcomes of this revisiting is nostalgia, understood broadly as a past-oriented, idiosyncratic, social, and bittersweet-but-overall-positive emotion that spans cultures (Sedikides & Wildschut, 2022). From a media psychological perspective, video game-induced nostalgia is especially compelling insofar as nostalgia can have therapeutic and analgesic properties—a comforting experience that has psychological and potentially even physical well-being benefits (Sedikides & Wildschut, 2018; Kersten et al., 2023).

The current chapter will provide an overview of the emerging psychological scholarship on nostalgia as induced by video games. Accordingly, much of the theory and research presented here is rooted in media psychology and mass communication scholarship, as these perspectives comprise our expertise and inform our understanding of nostalgia in video games. First, we provide a brief discussion of how one defines and specifies the types of games expected to elicit nostalgia (such as defining retrogames, Aycock, 2016; BBC, n.d.) as well as a summary of cultural and economic forces involved in gaming nostalgia (such as the preservation and/or remanufacture of seemingly classic games, Allen, 2021; Dyson, 2017). Next, we define nostalgia and discuss more specific definitions of nostalgia, such as the distinction between personal nostalgia (for one's own autobiographical memories) and historical nostalgia (as an impression or a sensemaking of prior eras; Natterer, 2014) and how this relates to nostalgia as a meaningful mediated experience (Bowman et al., 2023b; Daneels et al., 2021). Following, we present evidence from scholarship on the correlations between nostalgic video game experiences and short-term subjective well-being (summarized in Bowman & Wulf, 2023), and identify areas of future research and development necessary to further explore the robustness and stability of these relationships. We conclude with a discussion about the myriad psychological implications of gaming-induced nostalgia, from boosting entertainment as well as for improving subjective well-being. We extract from this research implications for game design—both on how to purposefully elicit nostalgia for current gaming experiences, and for how current gaming experiences might be expected to foster nostalgia far into the future.

## A brief note on defining retrogames

As noted in the introduction, video games have been a popular form of entertainment media since at least the mid-20th century. That said, defining what we consider what is or is not a retrogame is not so straightforward, given that the notion of "retro" is always relative to a point in time. As Gee (2019) argued:

> Does a game become retro after a certain number of years are passed? Is it when the game's hardware is no longer supported or produced? Or is it when its aesthetics are no longer mainstream? (p. 57).

Aycock (2018) further argues that another barrier to defining retrogames is that gaming technologies coexist and overlap with each other—we can see this for example in the release dates of home gaming consoles, such as the so-called 4th generation of consoles (e.g., Super Famicom/SNES and Sega Mega Drive/Genesis) surviving well into the 1990s, while 5th generation consoles (e.g., Sony's PlayStation) already released as of 1995 (BBC, n.d.). The shift from cartridge-based to CD-based game software brought with it fundamental shifts in the gaming experience, yet on consoles for which gamers of the time would have had equal access to.

That said, Gee (2019) provides a useful framework for considering retrogaming in terms of specific markers that could typify bygone gaming experiences. Examples could be games providing "three lives and health bar" and "high score" displays, both mechanics held over from coin-operated arcade games (also see Bowman et al., 2023b). In a similar vein, we can turn to Lewin's (2023) reporting that as of this writing, as many as 89% of all video games ever developed can no longer be played in their original form, thus suggesting that retrogames could be those that are endangered or even extinct. As it will become apparent later in this chapter, modern incarnations of retrogames might engage a "pastness" or flavor of these former experiences (see Grainge, 2000), perhaps as a way to preserve their essence, or to celebrate their unique mechanics when contrasted with modern gaming experiences.

All said, there is clear interest in retrogaming experiences–from the more than 30 million subscribers to the Nintendo Switch Online service that allows gamers access to historical games from the Nintendo catalogue (Allen, 2021) to the recent re-release of the Atari 2600+ game console capable of paying original Atari game cartridges (Atari, 2023). Others such as Dyson (2017) write about ongoing efforts to collect and preserve electronic games—perhaps as an effort to engage with a cultural memory of and appreciation for video games (Bowman et al., 2023b; Seremetakis, 1994).

## Nostalgia as a psychological phenomenon

Definitions of nostalgia are manifold and closely connected to the perspective that deals with the phenomenon. Etymologically, the word nostalgia derives from the Greek words for homecoming (νόστος; nostos) and pain (άλγος; algos). Most prominently, Homer's Odysseus was suffering ten years on his Odyssey to get home to his wife Penelope after the Trojan War. His memories of his wife, son, and homeland Ithaka, however, motivated him to keep fighting and continuing his journey to finally return home. From the perspective of (media) psychology, the definition of nostalgia derived by social psychologists appears essential for its application on gaming and (potential) well-being effects. In fact, Sedikides and colleagues (2015) define nostalgia as a "self-conscious, bittersweet but predominantly positive and fundamentally social emotion" (p. 190) that is triggered by reflection of fond memories.[1] Social psychological research following Sedikides and colleagues' (2015) definition of

1 Note that some theorists suggest the bittersweet nature reflects a negative consequence of nostalgia. For example, Impert and Rubin (2011) demonstrated a correlation between nostalgia and grief when remembering someone who has passed. However, others have shown how nostalgia can support the grieving process, suggesting the complexity of nostalgia as something that can be both positive and negative (Reid et al., 2021). Specific to video games, Yang & Liu (2017) found that escapism and nostalgia were negatively correlated with subjective well-being, which could be related to companion scholarship on time perspective in which past negative individuals could see nostalgic reverie as a painful experience (in contrast to past positive people; see Jankowski et al., 2020). Finally, from a sociological perspective, there is a tradition of scholarship on the negative and politically insidious implications of nostalgia–for example, those invoking a nostalgic mood (Grainge, 2000) to glorify the past (such as *Making [Thing] Great Again*). An overview of these arguments applied to media scholarship is presented in Kalinina (2016).

nostalgia has uncovered its manifold functions since the early 2000s. Thereby, this view entails a paradigm shift, as nostalgia was previously dismissed for a long time as a predominantly neg-ative state, as kind of "homesickness," and was even classified as a disease in the 17th century (Hofer, 1688/1934; Sedikides et al., 2004).

Nostalgia is a so-called mixed emotion. While on the one hand, people look through symbolic rose-tinted glasses and valorize the memories as particularly positive, they also experience a certain melancholy in the certainty that things will never be the same again. Following Frijda's (2007) classification of emotions, Hepper and colleagues (2012) therefore argue that nostalgia should be understood as a mixed emotion due to the co-activation of positive and negative affect. Another comparable mixed emotion is poignancy, an emotional response to personally significant events (e.g., Ersner-Hershfield et al., 2008). Finally, Hepper and colleagues conduct a prototype analysis. In a series of seven studies in total, they ask participants about the features of nostalgia, categorize them, rank the importance of the features, and finally recategorize the features into central and peripheral features of nostalgia. Core features of nostalgia are personally meaningful memories of places, things, and people; positive affect such as happiness, and (rather peripheral) negative affect such as loss and fear. This prototype was validated across various cultural backgrounds (Hepper et al., 2014).

Existing research on nostalgia as a psychological phenomenon and mixed emotion has uncovered three fundamental psychological functions (cf. Sedikides et al., 2015): First, nostalgia takes on a meaning-making function (also referred to as existential function). Nostalgic people perceive more meaningfulness in their own lives and, at the same time, search less for meaning in their own lives (Routledge et al., 2011; 2012). In a 2010 study, Juhl and colleagues show that nostalgia can reduce the existential threat that is triggered when confronted with one's own mortality in the context of terror management theory.[2] Second, nostalgia fulfils a self-oriented function that supports the self. Nostalgic people have better access to their intrinsic self-concept, and have a better idea of what they are really like (Baldwin et al., 2015). They are more optimistic (Cheung et al., 2013), more confident, and more aware of their positive attributes (Baldwin & Landau, 2014, Vess et al., 2012). Finally, nostalgia's social function is mirrored in research suggesting that nostalgic people feel more connected to other people in their lives and, overall, less lonely (Wildschut et al., 2006; Zhou et al., 2008).

Most of the studies demonstrating these three functions of nostalgia have been researched using the so-called Event Reflection Task (ERT, Sedikides et al., 2015).

2 Terror management theory (Greenberg et al., 1986) argues that when people are made aware of their own mortality, they cope with this anxiety by engaging and sustaining cultural beliefs, and finding other ways to boost self-esteem. Nostalgia could function as a buffer by reminding people of their broader life's meaning (also see Greenberg & Arndt, 2012).

Following this approach, there are two experimental groups: While one group is asked to write an essay about a common everyday situation, the other is instructed to recall an experience that makes them nostalgic. While ERT is a methodologically clean way to investigate these kinds of effects, nostalgia in everyday life is rarely triggered via such an artificial instruction. Thus, Wulf and colleagues (2018) argue that media content that reminds people of individual and fond memories can trigger similar effects. Such media can be, for example, specific songs that were playing at a certain, meaningful event (a wedding, anniversary, graduation party, first kiss, etc.) or movies that are connected to meaningful memories (the first movie you went to with parents, a franchise of beloved superheroes or cartoon characters from one's childhood). Indeed, many studies attest that a wide range of (media) stimuli can trigger nostalgia, ranging from visual (photos and objects, Holbrook & Schindler, 1996) and auditory (songs; Barrett et al., 2010), olfactory (smells; Reid, Green, Wildschut, & Sedikides, 2014) and gustatory stimuli (tastes; Supski, 2013). Initial studies have also attempted to elicit nostalgia via haptic stimuli, such as the specific shape of video game controllers (Bowman et al., 2023a; 2023b).

## Video games, nostalgia, and well-being

Through a rose-tinted heads-up display, video games, like other forms of media content, have the propensity to trigger nostalgia (Neimeyer, 2014) by transporting gamers back in time, serving as "[digital] time machines" (Wulf et al., 2018, p. 61). Literature has identified ways in which nostalgia can be triggered through video games. One way nostalgia can be triggered is through recall of an individual's own memories. This can be prompted after watching a video game trailer from one's childhood (Natterer, 2014), or writing about a memorable gaming experience from a bygone era (Wulf et al. 2020). Research has also demonstrated that nostalgia can be triggered through game play of either a modern version of nostalgic content (e.g., playing POKÉMON GO (Niantic, 2016); Bonus et al., 2018) or nostalgia can be induced by playing older nostalgic content (e.g., playing SUPER MARIO BROS. (Nintendo, 1985) on the NES Classic; Bowman et al., 2023a). The prior citations are examples of an individual's own personal (nostalgic) experiences (Bowman et al., 2023b); and playing nostalgic content allows individuals to connect with their past and play games from their childhood (Harborth & Pape, 2020). However, other forms of nostalgic memories may not be linked to an individual's personal lived experiences, rather a preference for media of a certain historical (nostalgic) time period (Natterer, 2014).

Historical nostalgia may be induced by referring to the culture and media of a different time period. This concept is represented in a variety of video game titles, where the design and narrative captures these bygone eras. THE BEATLES: ROCK

BAND (Harmonix, 2009) is one example of a documentary type game, which references the romanticized pop culture of the 1960s (Hodson, 2012). Others include FAR CRY 3: BLOOD DRAGON (Ubisoft Montreal, 2013), which borrows a "nostalgic mode" from 1980s science fiction action films (Sloan, 2015), and GONE HOME (The Fullbright Company, 2013), set in the 1990s in the US and using with period-accurate foods, soda cans, and clothing (Sloan, 2015). Video games offer a unique opportunity for individuals with no prior gameplay experience to feel a part of a prior generation (Bowman et al., 2022). This illustrates the diversity in which developers utilize nostalgia, as it can be used as a tool to reach a wider audience (Pearce, 2008). Using SUPER MARIO BROS. as an example, individuals will dedicate their resources to the demanding nature of video games (Bowman, 2018; 2021) to reconnect with their past (personal nostalgia) or to connect with a prior generation of gamers (historical nostalgia).

A synonymous finding between the aforementioned literature on personal and historical nostalgia is the positive influence that nostalgic content has on an individual, with regard to psychological well-being and subjective well-being. These positive effects on well-being are highlighted in the media-induced nostalgic contributions to the well-being model (MINCoW; Wulf et al., 2018) which stipulates that:

- Nostalgia has a direct influence on media experiences and outcomes, such as enjoyment and appreciation
- Nostalgia contributes directly to well-being through self-oriented, existential, and social functions
- Entertainment outcomes mediate the indirect effect nostalgia has on well-being

Video games research has tested some assumptions presented in the MINCoW model. Addressing the first assumption, Yang and Liu (2017) found a significant correlation between game play and enjoyment in POKÉMON GO. Ghazali et al. (2018) also discovered that enjoyment of POKÉMON GO influenced continued play. Research by Bonus et al. (2018) found that playing POKÉMON GO was associated with nostalgic feelings as well as friendship formation and intensification, which addresses the second assumption. Regarding the third assumption, research found that playing a nostalgic video game, such as POKÉMON GO, predicted eudaemonic (personally meaningful) entertainment experiences, which had an indirect effect on psychological well-being (such as personal flourishing; Wulf & Baldwin, 2020).

Previous research has identified a strong association between gaming-induced nostalgia and social connectedness. It has been found that individuals who played with guild members in WORLD OF WARCRAFT (Blizzard, 2004), would experience less loneliness and social anxiety online compared to the real world (Martončik & Lokša, 2016). Furthermore, individuals who played WORLD OF WARCRAFT CLASSIC had stronger feelings of nostalgia when they felt a higher sense of social presence

(Robinson & Bowman, 2021), which demonstrates the social role that nostalgia plays. Wulf et al. (2020) found that when participants recalled a personally nostalgic video gaming experience, memories often included time spent with family members or friends, which resulted in higher levels of optimism, self-esteem, and vitality. This demonstrated the positive effect of past social gaming memories, which increased levels of nostalgia, which in turn resulted in higher psychological and subjective well-being.

## Designing games with nostalgia in mind

To date, research into nostalgia in video games is comparatively light when we consider the 60-plus year history of the gaming medium, and the wealth of anecdotal evidence suggesting the cultural and economic appeal of retrogaming. Intuitively, it is clear that the audience for video games has aged along with the medium, and we can find a combination of seasoned gamers eager to replay their boards, screens, and worlds of yesterday. Just as well, we see newer gamers equally as eager to engage those seemingly bygone gaming experiences–to get a sense for earlier "eras" of video games as a way to more deeply engage with and experience the medium. From this nascent body of scholarship, we can already see paths forward that have implications for how games are imagined, engaged, experienced and enjoyed.

## Nostalgic mode and retrogaming design

Conversations around nostalgia in video games tend to focus solely on either bygone games and gaming technologies (such as the aforementioned *NES* home game console) or on releases of familiar and established gaming properties (such as the aforementioned POKÉMON and SUPER MARIO BROS.). These intellectual properties and trademarks have followings stemming from decades of gaming experience, and their re-releases serve as proxy indicators of their legacies–both for video games and for pop culture broadly. That said, there are numerous releases that engage with various features and attributes of older video games, while being based on entirely new characters, narratives, and intellectual properties. Grainge (2000) involves the notion of *nostalgic mode*—borrowing from Jameson's (1991) notes on postmodernism—to explain an aesthetic engagement with nostalgic content. Here, it is possible for the "look and feel" of older video games to be engaged by recreating elements common to the medium. Schrey (2014) talks specifically about how media cultures might celebrate the uniqueness of engaging with the limitations of media technologies–in older video games, this might include pixel art and animation (Makai, 2018) as well as chiptune music from 8-bit and 16-bit processors

(Driscoll & Diaz, 2009). Such animations and sounds were standard for their eras, but when used in modern video games evoke a sense of "pastness" for video games as a medium. For Grainge, (2000), such engagement can be understood as "an increasing semiotic awareness of the textuality of the past." To this end, we can consider the popularity of the aptly named "Metroidvania" genre of video games.[3] Such games borrow mechanics from a seemingly bygone genre of video games in the two-dimensional action platformer, often featuring pixel graphics and similar music while encouraging players to explore and "board by board"—often visiting older parts of the game map once newer abilities and skills are discovered (see Figure 1). Such a game genre is somewhat outdated in the era of sensory immersive and persistent online three-dimensional worlds, in which gamers can move in near-complete 360-degree space to navigate crafted environments from a first-person perspective. Games such as 9 YEARS OF SHADOWS (Halberd Studios, 2023) engage the "nostalgic mode" of games from the late 1980s and early 1990s, while presenting game content that is wholly original.[4] The game was highly regarded as a "bright spot among Metroidvanias" (Cart, 2023), with a statement somewhat suggesting a potential market saturation of the genre. In a similar vein, Oliveira et al. (2020) noted that Metroidvania games are an increasingly popular focus of indie game developers. Among many reasons for this could be a combination of the experiences of these developers (many of whom "grew up" on Metroidvania-type games) to a broader cultural appreciation for a style of gaming paradoxically novel and unique to contemporary gamers.

It is clear that Metroidvania games are popular, yet it is less clear as to whether and how these games might be experienced as *nostalgic* video games experiences. Open questions to consider might be the extent to which established gamers experience a sense of personal nostalgia for the nostalgic mode presented in these games—perhaps being reminded of bygone gaming experiences. Likewise, we could further investigate the extent to which younger gamers experience historical nostalgia for these games—perhaps engaging them with a sense of appreciation for the gaming as a whole (somewhat replicating Bowman et al., 2023b). Moreover, it could be that other gameplay mechanisms of "older" video games are likely to be engaged via nostalgic modes, given that retrogames are a relative categorization that

---

3 The namesake of this genre of games is a portmanteau of two classic video game properties in METROID (Nintendo, 1987) and CASTLEVANIA (Konami, 1986); see Oliveira et al. (2020).

4 Notably, games such as 9 YEARS OF SHADOWS are also representative of more diverse and inclusive voices not commonly featured in the history of video game development. For this game, the developer Halberd Studios is based in the Zapopan district of Guadalajara, Jalisco, Mexico (more information: https://www.halberdstudios.com/). The game's aesthetics were further inspired by anime programs such as SAILOR MOON and SAINT SEIYA (for more details, see https://steamcommunity.com/app/1402120/discussions/0/3825284962834862035/).

depends on the player's own experiences. Developers and researchers alike are encouraged to consider defining and delineating between various nostalgic notes, as understanding how engaging a nostalgic mode positively or negatively influences player experiences would be useful for developers who might seek out other "bygone" gaming aesthetics to emulate (also noted by Gee, 2019).

*Figure 1: The game map from 9 Years of Shadows (Halberd Studios, 2023). This level design is a standard feature of classic video games from the 1980s and early 1990s, when the technology did not allow for extensive and sensory immersive three-dimensional worlds. Instead, players navigated interconnected "rooms" with an end goal of unlocking all rooms and finding various objects and skills*

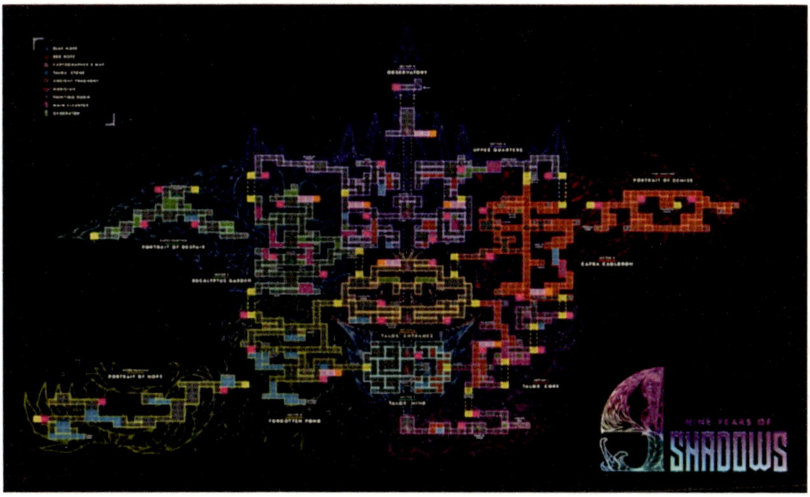


Map used with permission of Halberd Studios

## Video games and parent-child relationships

In prior research on video games and nostalgia, Wulf et al. (2020) came across the following comment shared by one of their survey participants: "My dad died when I was 10, so [playing MARIO KART with him] is one of my best memories of him." Although the quote was unique in terms of its sombreness, it was typical of more than 25% of the nostalgic memories shared by players (and nearly half of the memories which individuals were asked to discuss were social memories). These data reflect recent industry reports. In the United States, for example, the Entertainment Software Association has consistently reported a high degree of parent-child gaming, from around 67% in their 2017 report (ESA, 2017) to 76% as of their 2023 report (ESA, 2023). Active parental mediation strategies in which parents help their children understand and engage with on-screen content through the co-play of video games are correlated with more positive and effective family communication (Jiow et al., 2017; Wang et al., 2018). Likewise, research into nostalgia as an autobiographical notion suggests that connecting and engaging with meaningful others, such as family, is especially relevant for memories that trigger nostalgia (Abeyta et al., 2015, also see Hepper et al., 2012). Taken as a whole, this research suggests that, along with the short-term benefits of parent-child video gaming for encouraging healthy family communication styles, these shared social entertainment experiences are precisely the sort that parents and their children are likely to cherish later in life.

Related to this, we can also consider other ways in which parents might share their own prior gaming experiences with their children. In writing about nostalgia and well-being, Bowman and Wulf (2023) came across a social media post in a retrogames-focused subreddit in which a person discussed the experience of stumbling across their parent's old video game save file from LEGEND OF ZELDA: OCARINA OF TIME (Nintendo, 1998).[5] The post kicked off several threads of conversation about the curiosity and novelty of engaging in what could be perceived as a highly personal and private experience–video game files could be seen as an extension of one's self in digital worlds, for many of the reasons previously stated. Media broadly can serve an important part of self-identity (for example, music and adolescent identity; North & Hargreaves, 2006) and likewise, sharing those self-relevant artefacts is yet another way that parents engage children, and how children might make sense of their parents' experience and identities. Game developer Jesse Schell has written about the notion of "persistent avatars" that might follow a player throughout the lifetime (MCV Staff, 2010), and already we can see this in games such as WORLD OF WARCRAFT, where some players have had active avatars (and the associated save files with those characters' progress) for nearly 30 years since the game's release in 2005. The paucity of research on sharing these potentially deep, meaningful, and idiosyncratic personal save files across generations is ripe for future study.

## Sense of place and digital locations

Another area ripe for exploration would be how players might form attachments to the various locations from their own video game history. Borrowing from cultural geography, the concept of *sense of place* (SoP) explains the idiosyncratic and interpersonal connections that one feels for self-referential locations. As defined by Tuan

---

5 The post is shared with permission of the original poster: https://www.reddit.com/r/n64/comments/y7oda7/using_my_dads_old_ocarina_save_file/

(1975), "to know a place fully means both to understand it in an abstract way and to know it as one person knows another" (Tuan, 1975, p. 152). Relph (1976) followed in suggesting that sense of place forms as a combination of our familiarity with, experiences in, and *genius loci* that we feel for spaces; Hauge (2007) further argues that sense of place is critical to our sense of identity.

Although SoP has been studied extensively with respect to physical locations, there is emerging evidence that digital places can also facilitate SoP in ways that are associated with nostalgic memories. Turner and Turner (2006) recreated museum exhibits in virtual reality systems, and participants remarked how their engagement with those exhibits reminded them of childhood visits to museums and other cultural exhibits with family and friends. Directly in video games, Bowman et al. (2020) found that after two months playing FALLOUT 76, players began to foster SoP for West Virginia (the US state rendered digitally in-game)–in particular, players not from West Virginia saw a steady increase in SoP on par with those players native to the region. Later work by Bowman, Vanderwelle et al. (2023) examined ASSASSIN'S CREED games and again found that engaging with those games fostered SoP for various historical locations (such as London and Paris). Few studies have looked at the relationships between video game locations and nostalgia (cf. Robinson & Bowman, 2021), but it would stand to reason that part of the appeal of retrogames would be a yearning to re-engage important and self-referential game locations for which players might well have spent 10s to 100s of hours of their formative years engaging with.

## Conclusion and future directions

Video games are a global economic and cultural mainstay, with a nearly 60-year history of engaging and delighting players by taxing their cognitive, emotional, physical, and social resources. Games are played across cultures and across the lifespan, and bygone gaming experiences leave lasting impressions–the games of yesterday serve as wellsprings of nostalgic reverie today, and the games of today have the potential to serve as nostalgic referents for tomorrow.

## References

Abeyta, A. A., Routledge, C., Roylance, C., Wildschut, T., & Sedikides, C. (2015). Attachment-related avoidance and the social and agentic content of nostalgic memories. *Journal of Social and Personal Relationships*, 32, 406–413 http://dx.doi.org/10.1177/0265407514533770

Allen, J. (2021, November 8). *Nintendo Switch Online has 32 million subscribers according to Nintendo*. NME. Retrieved from https://www.nme.com/news/gaming-news/

nintendo-switch-online-has-32million-subscribers-according-to-nintendo-3090023

Atari. (2023). Atari 2600+. *Atari*. Retrieved from https://atari.com/products/atari-2600-plus

Aycock, J. (2016). *Retrogame archeology: Exploring old computer games*. Springer. https://doi.org/10.1007/978-3-319-30004-7

Barrett, F. S., Grimm, K. J., Robins, R. W., Wildschut, T., Sedikides, C., & Janata, P. (2010). Music-evoked nostalgia: affect, memory, and personality. Emotion, 10, 390–403. https://doi.org/10.1037/a0019006

BBC (n. d.). The 8 generations of video game consoles. BBC. Retrieved from https://www.bbc.co.uk/archive/the-8-generations-of-video-game-consoles/zvcjkty

Baldwin, M., Biernat, M., & Landau, M. J. (2015). Remembering the real me: Nostalgia offers a window to the intrinsic self. Journal of Personality and Social Psychology, 108, 128–147. https://doi.org/10.1037/a0038033

Baldwin, M., & Landau, M. J. (2014). Exploring nostalgia's influence on psychological growth. *Self and Identity*, 13, 162–177. https://doi.org/10.1080/15298868.2013.772320

Blizzard Entertainment. (2004). WORLD OF WARCRAFT [Microsoft Windows and macOS]. Blizzard Entertainment.

Bonus, J. A., Peebles, A., Mares, M.-L., & Sarmiento, I. G. (2018). Look on the Bright Side (of Media Effects): Pokémon Go as a Catalyst for Positive Life Experiences. *Media Psychology, 21*(2), 263–287. https://doi.org/10.1080/15213269.2017.1305280

Bowman, N. D. (2018). The demanding nature of video game play. In N.D. Bowman (Ed.), *Video games: A medium that demands our attention* (pp. 1–24). Routledge.

Bowman, N. D. (2021). Interactivity as demand: Implications for interactive media entertainment. In C. Klimmt & P. Vorderer (Eds.), *Oxford handbook of media entertainment*. Oxford University Press.

Bowman, N. D., Banks. J., Rittenour, C. (2020). Country roads through 1s and 0s: Sense of place for and recollection of West Virginia following long-term engagement with Fallout 76. *Technology, Mind, and Behavior*, 1(1). https://psycnet.apa.org/doi/10.1037/tmb0000001

Bowman, N. D., & Wulf, T. (2023). Nostalgia in video games. *Current Opinions in Psychology*, 49. https://doi.org/10.1016/j.copsyc.2022.101544

Bowman, N. D., Vandewelle, A., Daneels, R., Lee, Y., & Chen. S. (2023). Animating a plausible past: Perceived realism and sense of place influence entertainment of and tourism intentions from historical video games. *Games & Culture*. https://doi.org/10.1177/15554120231162428

Bowman, N. D., Velez, J., Wulf, T., Breuer, J., Yoshimura, K., & Resignato, L. J. (2023a). That bygone feeling: Controller ergonomics and nostalgia in video game play. *Psychology of Popular Media, 12*(2), 147–158. https://doi.org/10.1037/ppm0000382

Bowman, N. D., Yoshimura, K., Bohaty, E., & Condis, M. (2023b). "Makes me feel like I was born in the wrong era": Gamer self-efficacy and appreciation, rather than controller type, correlate with historical nostalgia when playing a retrogame. *Psychology of Popular Media*. https://doi.org/10.1037/ppm0000492

Cart, B. (2023, April 21). '9 Years of Shadows' review: Symphony of light. *NPR*. Retrieved from https://www.npr.org/2023/04/21/1170862559/9-years-of-shadows-review-symphony-of-the-light-castlevania-metroidvania

Cheung, W.-Y., Wildschut, T., Sedikides, C., Hepper, E. G., Arndt, J., & Vingerhoets, J. J. M. (2013). Back to the future: nostalgia increases optimism. *Personality & Social Psychology Bulletin, 39*, 1484–1496. https://doi.org/10.1177/0146167213499187

Clement, J. (2023, June 15). Video game industry – statistics & facts. *Statista*. Retrieved from https://www.statista.com/topics/868/video-games/#topicOverview

Crogan, P., & Kennedy, H. (2009). Technologies between games and culture. *Games & Culture, 4*(2), 107–114. https://doi.org/10.1177/1555412008325482

Daneels. R., Bowman, N. D., Possler, D., & Mekler, E. (2021). The 'eudaimonic experience': A scoping review of the concept in digital games research. *Media & Communication, 9*(2). https://doi.org/10.17645/mac.v9i2.3824

Driscoll, K. & Diaz, J. (2009). Endless loop: A brief history of chiptunes. *Transformative Works and Cultures*. 2(1). https://doi.org/10.3983/twc.2009.096

Dyson, J. P. C. (2017). Collecting, preserving, and interpreting the history of electronic games. *American Journal of Play, 10*(1). Retrieved from https://eric.ed.gov/?id=EJ1166783

Entertainment Software Association (2017). *Essential facts about the computer and video game industry*. ESA. Retrieved from https://www.theesa.com/wp-content/uploads/2021/03/ESA_EssentialFacts_2017.pdf

Entertainment Software Association (2023). *Essential facts about the U.S. video game industry*. ESA. Retrieved from https://www.theesa.com/2023-essential-facts/

Ersner-Hershfield, H., Mikels, J. A., & Sullivan, S. J. (2010). Poingnancy: mixed emotions in meaningful endings. *Journal of Personality, 94*, 158–167. https://doi.org/10.1037/0022-3514.94.1.158

Frijda, N. H. (2007). *The laws of emotion*. LEA.

Gee, D. (2019). Remixing retro: Preserving the "classic feeling". *Journal of the Japanese Association for Digital Humanities, 4*(1), 54–71. https://doi.org/10.17928/jjadh.4.1_54

Ghazali, E., Mutum, D. S., & Woon, M.-Y. (2019). Exploring player behavior and motivations to continue playing Pokémon GO. *Information Technology & People, 32*(3), 646–667. https://doi.org/10.1108/ITP-07-2017-0216

Grainge, P. (2000) Nostalgia and style in retro America: Moods, modes, and media recycling. *Journal of American Culture, 23*(1), 27–34. https://doi.org/10.1111/j.1537-4726.2000.2301_27.x

Greenberg, J., & Arndt, J. (2012). Terror management theory. In P. A. M. Van Lange, A. W. Kruglanski, & E. T. Higgins (Eds.), *Handbook of theories of social psychology* (pp. 398–415). Sage. https://doi.org/10.4135/9781446249215.n20

Greenberg, J., Pyszczynski, T., & Solomon, S. (1986). The causes of and consequences of a need for self-esteem: A terror management theory. In R. F. Baumeister (Ed.), *Public self and private self* (pp. 189–212). Springer-Verlag.

Halberd Studios. (2023). 9 YEARS OF SHADOWS. [Steam]. Halberd Studios.

Harborth, D., & Pape, S. (2020). How nostalgic feelings impact Pokémon Go players – integrating childhood brand nostalgia into the technology acceptance theory. *Behaviour & Information Technology, 39*(12), 1276–1296. https://doi.org/10.1080/0144929X.2019.1662486

Harmonix. (2009). THE BEATLES: ROCK BAND [Sony Playstation 3, Nintendo Wii, and Microsoft Xbox 360]. MTV Games.

Hauge, Å. L. (2007). Identity and place: A critical comparison of three identity theories. *Architectural Science Review, 50*(1), 44–51. https://doi.org/10.3763/asre.2007.5007

Hepper, E. G., Ritchie, T. D., Sedikides, C., & Wildschut, T. (2012). Odyssey's end: lay conceptions of nostalgia reflect its original Homeric meaning. *Emotion, 12*, 102–119. https://doi.org/10.1037/a0025167

Hepper, E. G., Wildschut, T., Sedikides, C., Ritchie, T., Yung, Y.-F., Hansen, N., Zhou, X. (2014). Pancultural nostalgia: Prototypical conceptions across cultures. *Emotion, 14*, 733–747. https://doi.org/10.1037/a0036790

History of Medicine, 2, 376–391 (Original work published 1688)

Hodson, J. (2021). *"When I'm sixty-four:" Beatles Rock Band and the commodification of nostalgia* [Other]. https://doi.org/10.32920/ryerson.14637966.v1

Holbrook, M. B., & Schindler, R. M. (1996). Market segmentation based on age and attitude toward the past: Concepts, methods, and findings concerning nostalgic influences on customer tastes. *Journal of Business Research, 37*, 27–39. https://doi.org/10.1016/0148-2963(96)00023-9

Impert, L., & Rubin, M. (2011). The mother at the glen: The relationship between mourning and nostalgia. *Psychoanalytic Dialogues, 21*(6), 691–706. https://doi.org10.1080/10481885.2011.629567/

Jameson, F. (1991). *Postmodernism, or the cultural logic of late capitalism*. Verso.

Jankowski, K. S., Zajenkowski, M., & Stolarski, M. (2020). What are the optimal levels of time perspectives? Deviation from the balanced time perspective-revisited (DBTP-r). *Psychological Belgica, 60*(1). https://doi.org/10.5334%2Fpb.487

Jenkins, H. (2006). Fans, bloggers, and gamers: Exploring participatory culture. *NYU Press*. http://dx.doi.org/10.18574/nyu/9780814743690.001.0001

Jiow H. J., Lim S.S., & Lin J. (2017). Level up! Refreshing parental mediation theory for our digital media landscape. *Communication Theory, 27*(3), 309–328. https://doi.org/10.1111/comt.12109

Juhl, J., Routledge, C., Arndt, J., Sedikides, C., & Wildschut, T. (2010). Fighting the future with the past: Nostalgia buffers existential threat. *Journal of Research in Personality, 44*, 309–314. https://doi.org/10.1016/j.jrp.2010.02.006

Kalinina, E. (2016). What do we talk about when we talk about media and nostalgia? *Medien & Zeit, 4*. Retrieved from https://medienundzeit.at/wp-content/uploads/2017/02/MZ-2016-4-online-ed.pdf#page=8

Kersten, M., & Cox, C. R. (2023). The past promotes the picture of health: Nostalgia as a resource for physical well-being. *Current Opinion in Psychology, 49*. https://doi.org/10.1016/j.copsyc.2022.101522

Konami. (1986). CASTLEVANIA. [Nintendo Entertainment System]. Konami.

Lewin, K. (2023, July 10). 87% missing: The disappearance of classic video games. *Video Game History Foundation*. Retrieved from https://gamehistory.org/87percent/

Makai, P. K. (2019). Video games as objects and vehicles of nostalgia. *Humanities, 7*(4), https://doi.org/10.3390/h7040123

Martončik, M., & Lokša, J. (2016). Do World of Warcraft (MMORPG) players experience less loneliness and social anxiety in online world (virtual environment) than in real world (offline)? *Computers in Human Behavior, 56*, 127–134. https://doi.org/10.1016/j.chb.2015.11.035

MCV Staff. (2010, November 10). Jesse Schell's persistent avatar vision. *MCV UK*. Retrieved from https://mcvuk.com/development-news/jesse-schells-persistent-avatar-vision/

Natterer, K. (2014). How and why to measure personal and historical nostalgic responses through entertainment media. *International Journal on Media Management, 16*(3), 161–180. https://doi.org/10.1080/14241277.2014.989567

Niantic. (2016). POKÉMON GO [iOS, Android]. Niantic.

Niemeyer, K. (2014). Introduction: Media and nostalgia. In K. Niemeyer (Ed.), *Media and nostalgia* (pp. 1–23). Palgrave Macmillan UK. https://doi.org/10.1057/9781137375889_1

Nintendo. (1985). SUPER MARIO BROS. [Nintendo Entertainment System]. Nintendo.

Nintendo. (1987). METROID. [Nintendo Entertainment System]. Nintendo.

Nintendo. (1998). LEGEND OF ZELDA: OCARINA OF TIME. [Nintendo 64]. Nintendo.

North, A. C., & Hargreaves, D. J. (2006). Music and adolescent identity. *Music Education Research, 1*(1), 75–92. https://doi.org/10.1080/1461380990010107

Oliveira, B. P., da Rocha Franco, A. dO., Franco de Silva, J. W., de Carvalho Gomes, F. A., & Rodrigues Maia, J. G. (2020). A framework for Metroidvania games. In *Proceedings of SBGames 2020*. Retrieved from https://www.researchgate.net/profile/Jose-Maia-4/publication/346540910_A_Framework_for_Metroidvania_Games/links/5fc67deda6fdccfea3f0770d/A-Framework-for-Metroidvania-Games.pdf

Pearce, C. (2008). The Truth About Baby Boomer Gamers: A Study of Over-Forty Computer Game Players. *Games and Culture, 3*(2), 142–174. https://doi.org/10.1177/1555412008314132

Reid, C. A., Green, J. D., Wildschut, T., & Sedikides, C. (2014). Scent-evoked nostalgia. *Memory, 23,* 157–166. https://doi.org/10.1080/09658211.2013.876048

Reid, C. A., Green, J. D., Short, S. D., Willis, K. D., Moloney, J. M., Collison, E. A., Wildschut, T. Sedikides, C. & Gramling, S. (2021). The past as a resource for the bereaved: Nostalgia predicts declines in distress. *Cognition and Emotion, 35*(2), 256–268. https://doi.org/10.1080/02699931.2020.1825339

Robinson, J. A., & Bowman, N. D. (2021). Returning to Azeroth: Nostalgia, sense of place, and social presence in World of Warcraft Classic. *Games & Culture, 17*(3), 421–444. https://doi.org/10.1177/15554120211034759

Routledge, C., Arndt, J., Wildschut, T., Sedikides, C., Hart, C., Juhl, J., Scholtz, W. (2011). The past makes the present meaningful: Nostalgia as an existential resource. Journal of *Personality and Social Psychology, 101,* 638–652. https://doi.org/10.1037/a0024292

Routledge, C., Wildschut, T., Sedikides, C., Juhl, J., & Arndt, J. (2012). The power of the past: nostalgia as a meaning-making resource. *Memory, 20,* 452–60. https://doi.org/10.1080/09658211.2012.677452

Schrey, D. (2014). Analogue nostalgia and the aesthetics of digital remediation. In K. Niemeyer (Ed.), *Media and nostalgia*. Palgrave Macmillan. https://doi.org/10.1057/9781137375889_2

Sedikides, C., & Wildschut, T. (2018). Finding meaning in nostalgia. *Review of General Psychology, 22,* 48–61. https://doi.org/10.1037/gpr0000109

Sedikides, C., & Wildschut, T. (2022). Nostalgia across cultures. *Journal of Pacific Rim Psychology, 16*. https://doi.org/10.1177/18344909221091649

Sedikides, C., Wildschut, T., & Baden, D. (2004). Nostalgia: Conceptual issues and existential functions. In J. Greenberg, S. Koole, & T. Pyszczynski (Hrsg.), *Handbook of experimental existential psychology* (S. 200–214). Guilford Press.

Sedikides, C., Wildschut, T., Routledge, C., Arndt, J., Hepper, E. G., & Zhou, X. (2015). To nostalgize: Mixing memory with affect and desire. *Advances in Experimental Social Psychology, 51,* 189–273. https://doi.org/10.1016/bs.aesp.2014.10.001

Seremetakis, C. N. (1994). *The memory of the senses, part 1: Marks of the transitory.* Routledge.

Sloan, R. J. S. (2015). Videogames as remediated memories: Commodified nostalgia and hyperreality in Far Cry 3: Blood Dragon and Gone Home. *Games and Culture,* 10(6), 525–550. https://doi.org/10.1177/1555412014565641

Supski, S. (2013). Aunty Sylvie's sponge: Food making, cookbooks and nostalgia. *Cultural Studies Review, 19,* 28–49. Retrieved from http://epress.lib.uts.edu.au/journals/index.php/csrj/article/viewFile/3074/3419

The Fullbright Company. (2013). GONE HOME [Microsoft Windows]. The Fullbright Company

Tuan, Y.-F. (1975). Place: An experiential perspective. *The Geographical Review, 65*(2), 151–165. https://doi.org/10.2307/213970

Turner, P., & Turner, S. (2006). Place, sense of place, and presence. *Presence, 15*(2), 204–217. https://doi.org/10.1162/pres.2006.15.2.204

Ubisoft Montreal. (2013). FAR CRY 3: BLOOD DRAGON [Sony PlayStation 3, Microsoft Windows, and Microsoft Xbox 360]. Ubisoft.

Vess, M., Arndt, J., Routledge, C., Sedikides, C., & Wildschut, T. (2012). Nostalgia as a resource for the self. *Self and Identity, 11*, 273–284. https://doi.org/10.1080/15298868.2010.521452

Wang, B., Taylor, L., & Sun Q. (2018). Families that play together stay together: Investigating family bonding through video games. *New Media & Society, 20*(11), 4074–4094. https://doi.org/10.1177%2F1461444818767667

Wildschut, T., Sedikides, C., Arndt, J., & Routledge, C. (2006). Nostalgia: content, triggers, functions. *Journal of Personality and Social Psychology, 91*, 975–93. https://doi.org/10.1037/0022-3514.91.5.975

Wulf, T., & Baldwin, M. (2020). Being a kid again: Playing Pokémon Go contributes to wellbeing through nostalgia. *Studies in Communication and Media, 9*(2), 241–263. https://doi.org/10.5771/2192-4007-2020-2-241

Wulf, T., Bowman, N. D., Rieger, D., Velez, J. A., & Breuer, J. (2018). Video games as time machines: Video game nostalgia and retro gaming. *Media & Communication, 6*(2), 60–60. https://doi.og/10.17645/mac.v6i2.1317

Wulf, T., Bowman, N. D., Velez, J. A., & Breuer, J. (2020). Once upon a game: Exploring video game nostalgia and its impact on well-being. *Psychology of Popular Media, 9*(1), 83–95. https://doi.org/10.1037/ppm0000208

Wulf, T., Rieger, D., & Schmitt, J. B. (2018). Blissed by the past: Theorizing media-induced nostalgia as an audience response factor for entertainment and well-being. *Poetics, 69*, 70–80. https://doi.org/10.1016/j.poetic.2018.04.001

Yang, C., & Liu, D. (2017). Motives matter: Motives for playing Pokémon Go and implications for well-being. *Cyberpsychology, Behavior, and Social Networking, 20*(1), 52–57. https://doi.org/10.1089/cyber.2016.0562

Zhou, X., Sedikides, C., Wildschut, T., & Gao, D.-G. (2008). Counteracting loneliness. On the restorative function of nostalgia. *Psychological Science, 19*, 1023–1029. https://doi.org/10.1111/j.1467-9280.2008.02194.x

# When Gamers Save Lives

## Qualitative Research on Gaming Communities, Peer Support and Mental Health

*Maude Bonenfant, Élisa Vial and Clara Lhotellier*

The gaming community is active and pervasive online. According to the canonical definition by Rheingold, "virtual communities are social aggregations that emerge from the Net when enough people carry on those public discussions long enough, with sufficient human feeling, to form webs of personal relationships in cyberspace" (1993, p. 5). While this definition gives sufficient criteria to define what a digital community is, there is not only one community of gamers nor one community per game. The core concept of "community" is abstract and boundaries between communities are blurred.

Nevertheless, the majority of gamers share a feeling of community. In other words, they are part of a group, sharing the same passion for one or multiple video games. Over time, gamers create social rules and share a common culture. This culture is based upon a specific vocabulary, inside jokes, past stories, particular ways of greeting, etc. The acquisition of this knowledge is structured through implicit social rules that tell the individual how to act within the group. Participation in the community nurtures a sense of belonging according to, for instance, years of experience, performance, and involvement. This social glue can be strong and be a big part of individuals' social life.

Even though the community is strictly speaking "imagined" (Anderson, 1983), the effects of a sense of belonging are well and truly real. They materialize through members' engagement. For instance, time commitment is a criterion used to judge involvement in the community. Playing, being informed about games, training, communicating on social media, and creating content can be perceived as an emotional involvement toward the game and the community. Social involvement materializes through welcoming new members, resources, and information sharing, or even peer support.

In general, peer support is a process of mental health recovery. It involves the intervention of people who have dealt with a mental disorder and have now learned to live with or overcome it. The core of peer support is a deep knowledge of certain troubles based on their own experience. Peer helpers can be trained or not and offer support to those who ask for it. Peer support used to be an alternative to psychiatric hospitals and other manifestations of the institutionalization and medicalization of mental health (Fortuna et al., 2022).

Nowadays, distinct types of peer support can be differentiated. Recent research highlights the diversity of peer support mechanisms, such as self-help groups, peer-delivered services, peer-run or operated services, peer partnerships, peer employees, and internet support groups (Fortuna et al. 2022). Digital peer support is not new (Fortuna et al., 2019). But with the COVID-19 pandemic, this type of mutual aid has grown (Fortuna et al., 2020). Many formal services have had difficulties adapting, showing shortcomings in digital peer support (Merchant et al., 2022). However, untrained people do lead digital peer support. They are active on social media, such as Facebook groups (Naslund et al., 2016b, 2018), forums (Mertan et al., 2020), comment sections (Frohlich et al., 2012), and chats (O'Leary et al., 2018). People disseminate information (Griffith et al., 2015; Mertan et al., 2020), promote events, and share fundraising opportunities for mental health groups (Bender et al., 2011). More simply, moral support is based on sharing stories (Chou et al., 2011; Frohlich et al., 2012; Naslund et al., 2014; Sangeorzan et al., 2019). Conversations appear on social media, for exam-ple under hashtags on X (formerly Twitter) (Berry et al., 2017). These digital discussions reach many people (Naslund, 2016a) and even target individuals without mental health issues.

Despite its essential role in good mental health, few studies deal with peer support in video game settings. In the cases where video games are discussed, peer support is mainly studied through the prism of the mentor/disciple relationship (Ahmad et al., 2010; Nardi, 2006; Rusk et al., 2020; Simon et al., 2009). Practiced by more than 3 billion individuals (techjury.net/blog/how-many-gamers-are-there/), video games are nevertheless essential for understanding how individuals offer or receive help from their peers, but also how gaming and communication platforms influence the organization of this peer support. This study aims to document the phenomenon of peer support in video game contexts and its role in gamers' mental health based on the experiences of the main actors, namely gamers, moderators, and other stakeholders.

The disciplinary field of this study is communication and more precisely game studies with a qualitative approach using semi-structured interviews (69 persons). From a social constructivist perspective, the study aims to understand how gamers perceive mutual aid and peer support within their gaming community. It is not a question of describing objective reality, but rather the way in which individuals have experienced this reality and talk about it. The study aims to report their words by identifying the general meaning and recurrences between the experiences in order to establish a general portrait of the phenomenon.

As a first step, we will explain (1.) the methodological approach used in this research. After that, we will present the results while putting them in perspective alongside other research. (2.) We will first emphasize that a sense of belonging to a community reduces feelings of isolation, which is the premise for peer-to-peer support's contribution to good mental health. (3.) Subsequently, we will look more precisely at how video games and communication tools influence the structuring of communities and peer support between gamers. Finally, we will show the positive aspects of this mutual aid between gamers. However, there are also (4.) some limitations: a critical look at peer support in a video game context yields plausible solutions so that gamers can really save lives.

## Methodological approach

Previous studies have not explored peer support in the video game context from a specific mental health angle. We, therefore, chose a qualitative exploratory approach. This research aims to document the phenomenon without a preliminary hypothesis. We want to explore the prevalence and forms of peer support among gaming communities. To do this, questioning people involved in gaming communities was deemed to be the best method to gain a general understanding of the situation. We conducted semi-structured interviews between 30 and 90 minutes by videoconference. They were recorded, transcribed verbatim, and then the recordings were destroyed. We assigned pseudonyms to each interview according to a specific nomenclature.

We conducted a total of 69 interviews. Recruits included gamers from 13 years old and older, parents of underage gamers, adult gamers, coordinators of informal or official peer support organizations, professional helpers, Discord moderators, and streamers. They were all French-speaking and lived mainly in Quebec (Canada). We recruited through several channels, such as Facebook, LinkedIn, Twitch and Discord groups, direct solicitations, indirect solicitations via people responsible for self-help groups or peer-support organizations, and by word-of-mouth. We established a socio-demographic questionnaire on LimeSurvey and 59 people responded. The majority of people were between 18 and 39 years old (91%) and, more particularly, between 25 and 34 (59%). Most respondents were men (61%), while 34% were women, 3.3% were non-binary people, and 1.7% didn't identify with the previous categories. Also, among the respondents, nearly 86.4% were white, 6.8% were indigenous, 1.7% were Latin American or Caribbean, 1.7% were Chinese or Sino-descendant, and the remaining identified with other origins. Nearly 22% of respondents had a community college degree, and 67% had a university degree. 64% of respondents were in a relationship, 7% were married, and 27% were single.

The games played by respondents were mainly shooting games, action role-playing games, and management games (concerning more than half of the responses). The most played games by participants were *WORD OF WARCRAFT* (2004, Blizzard Entertainment), *LEAGUE OF LEGENDS* (2009, Riot Games), *COUNTER-STRIKE* (2000, Valve), *CALL OF DUTY* (2003, Activision), and *OVERWATCH* (2016, Blizzard Entertainment). Gamers were mostly PC gamers (74.6%), followed by home consoles (17%) and less significantly cellular and tablet console gamers (3.4%), and 1.6% didn't answer.

Following the transcription of interviews, we coded the verbatims on Nvivo using thematic and content analysis, i.e., by extracting the meaning of the interviewees' remarks according to specific categories. An analysis grid was thus created iteratively between categories predetermined before the interview and categories that emerged following the interviews inductively. The main categories of analysis were the personal portrait of the gamer, interpersonal relationships, and the relationship between the gamer and video games. For this chapter, we were particularly interested in the category of interpersonal relationships. This category comprises creating a social network, mutual aid, toxicity, problematic social relationships, and gamers' motivations to help others. For this paper, these categories have been reorganized into three sections: (2.) sense of belonging to a community and reduction of isolation as a factor in good mental health, (3.) organization of the gaming community to promote peer help and good mental health and, finally, (4.) current limitations of peer support in video game settings.

## Sense of belonging and reduced isolation as a factor in good mental health

Video games and digital communication platforms play a significant role in socialization (Taylor, 2006; Castronova, 2008; Pearce, 2011; etc.). Among adolescent men, online video games are one of the preferred ways to build strong friendships (Lenhart et al., 2015). Generally speaking, gamers often start playing online with friends they met offline (Lenhart, 2018). In his study, Sundberg, citing Domahidi, Festl, and Quandt (2014), demonstrates that online gamers tend to make friends more quickly online. Based on the work of Schiano et al. (2011) and Martončik et al. (2016), Sundberg adds that massively multiplayer online role-playing games (MMORPGs) are games that strengthen the bonds that bind people together, especially those encountered offline.

> You can make friendships [in gaming communities]. A person may not have any friends in real life, always stays at home and tells themself that they want to start playing in groups online. (CM_RT1_H)

> There are people I've played with for ten years that I've never met. Only after ten years did we see each other for the first time. They have been like best friends since childhood. (CM_TF1_H)

The presence of other gamers in the game can play a positive role by reducing social isolation (Halbrook et al. 2019). Lockdowns related to the global COVID-19 pandemic have demonstrated the importance of online video games in maintaining an active social life and good mental health (Homo Ludens, 2021; Lewis et al., 2021; Zhu, 2020; Barr et al., 2021; Bengtsson et al., 2021; Johannes et al. 2020). The World Health Organization even launched the *Play Apart Together* campaign in 2020 to encourage people to have an active social life while remaining physically isolated. The relaxation, stimulation, and feeling of commitment that playing the game provides are conducive to exchange between gamers and, ultimately, a better mental balance.

> He [a viewer on Twitch] told me that during the Covid pandemic, I really helped him with my streams. They [gamers on Discord groups] think, "I'm going to share my day, and there's bound to be someone to answer me, and I'll feel less alone." Many people have difficulty with socialization. They don't have many friends, live on rejection, and have little self-esteem. But at the [official peer support organism], we reinforce positive behaviors, we congratulate ourselves, and we respect each other. (CM_MZ1_F)

Several features offered by the games aim to put gamers in contact, whether they know each other or not outside the gaming context: friend lists, matchmaking, in-game chats, or guilds. Types of games based on lasting connections, like MMORPGs, are particularly effective at producing a sense of belonging. A previous study (Bonenfant et al., 2018) demonstrated how the rules and features of the MMORPG GUILD WARS II (2012, ArenaNet) promote friendly social relationships where mutual aid is so encouraged that it becomes normalized within the community. On the contrary, a multiplayer online battle arena (MOBA) game like LEAGUE OF LEGENDS (Riot Games, 2009), for example, overvalues individual performances, thus leading to competition between gamers within the same team. Few acts of mutual aid are observed in play since agonistic relationships quickly become antagonistic, and toxic acts can occur between gamers.

However, highly competitive games, such as MOBAs, Battle Royale games, or shooters, remain popular. They stimulate a massive amount of gamers to communicate on various platforms, produce content, and maintain an active community outside of games. Communication tools, such as Discord, and social media, such as Twitch, make it possible to meet gamers, chat, maintain relationships, and even develop friendships (Lenhart, A. et al. 2015; Sunberg, M. 2018; Domahidi, E. et al., 2014).

> For example, they [gamers] come to Twitch because they feel lonely. They don't want to play alone. With Twitch, they create a community naturally, and they can exchange on topics. It acts as a first line, a social safety net. (CM_MZ1_F)

> You can create links on these digital social media, including a person who does not have many friends, is still at home, and would like to play in a group. (CM_RT1_H)

> One of the best things that can happen is the sense of belonging. Isolation is the worst thing. Streaming tends to break social isolation, and it helps for a while. (CM_PP1_F)

Whether the gamers are close friends or not, the video game is a way for some to escape isolation and break a negative spiral. Gamers log in, knowing that someone will be there to interact with them. In more established and closer communities, gamers can directly write to each other to offer "a session" where gamers find themselves online without necessarily playing the same game but always listening to each other. In some cases, gamers join different online communities in order to get moral support.

> I believe that video games are an escape, whether solo or not, a way to live a different adventure, to forget their daily life or problems for a time. Playing online in a group is a way to socialize and to have human contact. Even if it's virtual, it's still human contact; it's still a great way to break the isolation. (CM_PP1_F)

Many gamers are regularly connected to Discord, leaving a channel of communication open almost constantly. Gamers highly regard this communication tool, as the company promotes and fosters a positive environment thanks to strict regulations and an organized ecosystem. Gamers feel safe to exchange on Discord. Whether in-game or on other online platforms, all these communication tools promote the networking of individuals, the creation of superficial or deep connections, and a sense of belonging to a group through social relationships maintained over time.

> When someone says they're not feeling well, eight people will want to help. Sometimes it is clumsy and the right resources are not given. But, everyone wants to help. Once they are in a community, they really feel that they belong because they want to help each other. [...] Whenever someone is not well, someone will respond. A helper can offer to talk privately or on the chat when live. (CM_AB2_F)

A community of gamers creates a strong sense of belonging, as they have a shared passion. Common interests promote the creation of connections, sometimes intense, and facilitate exchanges since they allow gamers to understand each other and to offer help. There is a real benevolence regarding the need not to feel alone and to feel understood.

Nevertheless, video games still get bad press among non-gamers, and the stigmatization of gamers reinforces this sense of understanding between them. This feeling of stigma becomes a pole of social recognition and a motivating engine within gaming communities and allows for positive reinforcement. The empathy created within communities, provoked by mutual aid, similar experiences, and a shared passion, thus makes it possible to repeat a vital pattern that plays a crucial role in peer support. Gamers who have experienced some form of mutual aid in-game or through different communication platforms will tend to reproduce this pattern. All these elements make it possible to strengthen this sense of belonging.

> We have a community that comes back frequently. These people have a heavy past but a big heart to help others [...]. I think it's beautiful because without knowing what to do, they use their own emotional experience to help and encourage each other and take the positive out of it. (CM_AB3_F)

Through this sense of community, gamers can create bonds of trust, leading to confidence, mutual aid, and support. Instead of hindering emotional relationships between gamers, pseudonymity can allow individuals to communicate more freely. In their work, Andalibi and Flood (2021) demonstrate that anonymity seems to be a factor in socialization and opening up to others. Interacting via an avatar while playing facilitates relationships in some peer support contexts. For these people, the exchange and sincerity of online and face-to-face meetings have the same value. For some gamers, exchanging online thus becomes a context conducive to trust and relaxation.

> I think it's positive [online relationships], especially for isolated people. And then many young people have more friends online, it's essential to have safe places to express themselves (CM_AB3_F)

> The distance created by the screen makes it more comfortable. You can trust and confide in someone you're sure you won't meet at school or work. You can tell them what's going on in your life without having any impact (CM_X10_H)

A kind of reassuring ambiance settles in, accentuated by distance and pseudonymity. Whether due to shyness, shame, or for other reasons, face-to-face communication can be difficult for some, if not impossible. For example, for individuals from gender, racialized, and religious minorities, neuroatypical people or people living with a disability, or anyone who is socially stigmatized, interconnecting through an avatar can be a social facilitator.

> I have a team of moderators that is diverse. There are people from the LGBTQ+ community from various backgrounds and ages, and all this makes people feel comfortable because they know it's a safe space (CM_MZ1_F)

In his study, Sundberg (2018) demonstrated that online video games help reduce loneliness in casual and regular gamers who are on the autism spectrum. Gamers on the spectrum tend to have more friends through online video games than people on the spectrum who do not play.

> Talking behind a screen helps greatly. You can say things you wouldn't have said in person. I'm someone who is slightly on the spectrum [of autism]. The rules are clear throughout the game, and I sincerely appreciate it. I understand everything. Even in terms of socializing through play, [social] conventions are more straightforward. It makes things easier for those struggling with face-to-face and interpersonal relationships (CM_X11_H)

In this context, where pseudonymity and clear social rules can help communication, people with mental health problems can benefit from participating in gaming communities.

## The gaming community promoting peer support and good mental health

The bonds of trust developed within the gaming community via gaming platforms, communication tools, and social media make peer support possible in the video game context. However, these devices influence the organization of mutual assistance between gamers. In addition to influencing the creation and maintenance of social relationships, gaming or communication platforms encourage a specific social organization, including a hierarchy based on the structure of the platforms. In the main games under consideration, rules and features define "roles" (the terminology of which may vary from game to game) that intersect with the skills and attitudes of each gamer to form a kind of "social class."

In general, to progress in the game, the different gamers form a team or guild, structured according to their strengths and weaknesses, to set a strategy. Depending on seniority, performance, knowledge, and personality, gamers occupy a role in the game while building their identity as a gamer.

However, these roles also influence the community's social hierarchy. For example, games like WORLD OF WARCRAFT divide roles into guilds with leaders, non-commissioned officers, regular members, and new gamers. These roles define not only the type of power of each gamer within the group, but also the rules of communication and how to interact. For example, the senior gamers will tend to gain the upper hand over newcomers who will have to be helped or socially rejected depending on the type of guild. In the case of a welcoming group for new gamers, a kind of mentoring is observable. This relationship is established within groups or informally between two gamers, one more experienced than the other.

> When I started playing Counter-Strike, I was lucky enough to get into a good team with good gamers and, especially one who was more mature. I must have been 14 years old. Thanks to him, I have never raged about a game, I never get angry. This person managed to focus us and help us improve. It had a big impact on me, even on my professional life. (GM_C2_H)

> My goal is to pass on my passion and help others advance in the game. Not every gamer wants to go pro, far from it. You have to find the balance: encourage people who want to perform, answer the questions of the curious gamers, and encourage them to experiment. (GM_C2_H)

This dynamic is particularly prevalent in MMORPGs (Ahmad et al., 2010; Nardi, B., 2006; Rusk, F. et al., 2020; Simon B. et al., 2009). This relationship initially aims at introducing the game and strategies. Nevertheless, this mentor relationship is then standardized and allows other types of mutual assistance, for example in the context of mental health.

In addition to mentoring, moderation is often self-organized within groups of gamers. Games offer tools that may or may not allow gamers to act against toxic behavior but, usually, the gamers decide the rules of social conduct. Some gamers then voluntarily guarantee moderate behaviors and become a model player to whom to address (Fortuna et al., 2022).

> Last year, I designed an anonymous complaint system that is now easier to understand and more accessible. In the community, there are more than 200 of us, so conflicts are normal and can be very intense. (CM_RT1_H)

Moreover, the social structure inside games is transferred to the out-game exchange platforms. In the same way, the roles in the game influence social hierarchy and relationships of mutual aid. For instance, the structure of Discord conditions the way the gamers interact with each other. At the top of the social pyramid are the servers' owners, then the channels' administrators, and the moderators present to maintain order between the primary members. Very invested and often connected, moderators ensure the proper functioning of the various channels, thus limiting overflows.

This moderation system is prominent in the practice of video games, such as *OVERWATCH*, and on different platforms, such as Discord and Twitch. Moderation and speaking space rules are essential for offline and online groups (Strand et al., 2020). They create a sense of community and prevent tensions (Kaplan et al., 2011).

They also lead to mutual aid relationships between gamers since moderators become a possible resource person for gamers in psychological distress. Many moderators thus see themselves becoming confidants, sometimes despite themselves and offer to listen while sharing their own experiences.

> I am very involved in gaming communities and not only with [a gamer group]. We really try to create a pleasant environment for everyone. In video games, we are there to have fun but unfortunately things happen, and we do not see everything. We are trying to stem that in our community [...]. That's why I proposed myself as president. I have a sense of belonging to this community, which made me want to get involved. It's volunteer work, and we are intensely involved so that the environment is pleasant for all. (CM_RT1_H)

This normalization of moderation and mutual aid has repercussions on the entire community as various unofficial roles appear, especially within Discord channels. For example, some members, perceived as members with a higher degree of engagement within the community or as informal moderators, are connected almost constantly without having a fully defined role. Becoming a resource person, they are a link between moderators and grassroots members. They act as a "sentinel" to identify individuals in need, even those with suicidal tendencies.

> If you need to talk, you can call. We remain present because if we do not do it, people will not stay because they do not trust the community. They can leave and become solo gamers, and that's not what we want. (CM_RT1_H)

> The [Twitch] platform allows them [gamers] to live positively, and their role affords them value. One of our subscribers is a moderator and helps a lot, for example. [...] People on our Discord want to become sentinels. They undergo a short training to identify the different signs to look for and how to act in this kind of situation. We have social workers who are experts in these issues, but these volunteer members come to support our team » [...]

> Sometimes complex situations happen when stakeholders are not connected. Nevertheless, many of the helpers are there during the week and at night on Discord. We also have the sentinels trained to help identify people in distress. We are vigilant to avoid reproducing problematic situations (CM_AB3_F)

This self-organization around mental health has become normalized to the extent that gamers have created more or less official structures. These structures thus ensure a better response to requests for help and perpetuate a form of knowledge on peer support acquired within the community. The role of "street workers" is held by some who claim to be caregivers and promote peer support to help others.

> We have a list of resources in case of suicidal thoughts or drug addiction. I can enumerate them for 30 minutes. We offer these hotlines to allow them to seek help, but we cannot take them by the hand and force them to do anything because we are not there for that. (CM_RT1_H)

> Mainly, mutual aid occurs in the chat. In the Discord channels, people continue speaking, exchanging, and helping each other with their own struggles. (CM_AB3_F)

An actual frontline social safety net is created within the games as gamers provide self-help. Listening to others and sharing experiences also promotes discussion and solidarity between gamers, who might then be more aware of the mental health issue and develop digital vigilance. Across platforms, gamers may be better able to recognize and intervene in cases of emotional distress. Some reflexes to adopt can be acquired, such as redirecting the person to professional support.

> I have noticed that even though there are resources such as crisis services, people seem reluctant to consult them because of a lack of trust. Sometimes, they need a little push. (CM_AB3_F)

> I don't know if we're on the frontline. That would be very flattering. We do all the management. *Aren't you well? Here's some help*. We want people not to feel like a simple number in a queue. We give resources, but we cannot do more. Moreover, many things in real life escape us. The only control we have is over the online community. (CM_RT1_H)

In addition, by valuing positive behaviors, gamers can better foster this healthy and positive environment (especially for new or younger gamers). Receiving help also encourages giving in return. It makes a positive difference, no matter how little it is.

To understand this virtuous loop of valuing positive behaviors within the community as a driver of group cohesion, we have established a diagram, "How peer support works for mental health in a gaming community" (see Figure 1). A sense of belonging stems from the concept of a gaming community. This sense of belonging implies recognition from peers and a willingness to get involved in the community. Within this community, self-organization structures social relations. But this organization is based on the social structures found in multiplayer games such as guilds or teams where a hierarchy is imposed through specific in-game roles. The same social pattern is reproduced on other platforms like Discord where the leaders have a higher position in Discord servers than other members. This self-organization makes it possible to create different social roles, from vigilance on the ground to structured help. This structured help begins with the members/regular players who act as sentinels, then the moderators who ensure a response to requests for help up to the people in charge who coordinate mutual aid. This structured organization thus forms a social safety net, understood here as a safe space to express oneself freely and find help. Talking about emotions or experiences can put oneself in a vulnerable situation, so one has to be safe to talk about it. In these safe spaces, members know that some gamers will listen to them and protect them from online harassment.

Finally, within the community, a phenomenon of prevention and awareness is taking place. Sharing individual experiences raises awareness on different topics among other members. It prevents toxic actions between players given the greater sensitivity towards others, but also it prevents violent acts towards oneself such as self-harm and suicide because help is provided. Being part of the same community, as we have seen before, gamers have a sense of belonging, and a dynamic of peer support is set up. Members provide listening and support, all in a moderated space. This sharing and support then reinforces the initial sense of belonging, creating a virtuous and dynamic circle of support between gamers within the communities.

The circle is thus closed since encouragement and positive communication based on respectful listening allow members of the community to create a stronger sense of belonging. The community is no longer simply based on a shared passion for video games but also on empathy and altruism. It promotes peer support through the development of mutual trust and a safe space to confide in and reinforce a sense of community.

*Figure 1: The virtuous loop of valuing positive behaviors.*

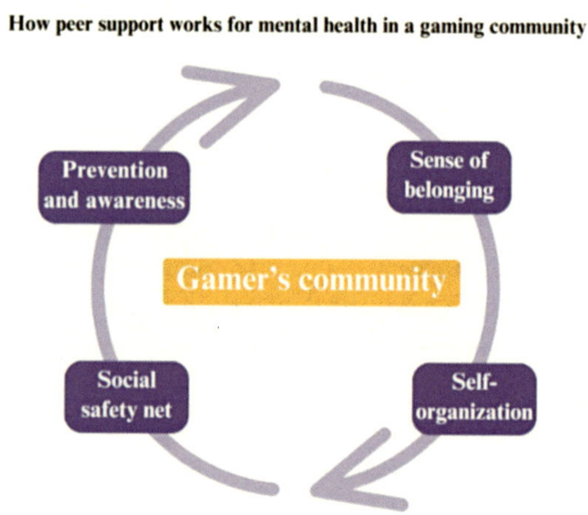

## The limits of peer support in video game contexts

Although self-help communities have many positive aspects and can be seen as an actual social safety net for people whose mental health may be fragile, peer support nevertheless has limitations, starting with the availability of peer helpers. Even though many Discord channels have volunteer responders to help gamers, the volume of people in distress is too large. In-game or out-game self-help platforms receive a high frequency of requests, but there is a limited number of peer helpers and a full schedule. Helpers are recruited voluntarily and have limited time to help.

> It isn't easy because we are not a 24-hour service, and we know that things happen outside of our services and opening hours. (CM_AB3_F)

> I do not do intervention during the stream because I am not equipped for that. […] We want to change the person's ideas but do not stop the stream to focus on the person. (CM_MZ1_F)

It often becomes impossible to provide immediate help. It is in this context that "ticket" systems emerge, in which each person can request a textual or video consultation with a helper. A "waiting line" is created. This structure is not adaptive if the person in distress may be in crisis and in need of immediate help. In addition, the ticket system does not provide for follow-up of people since each meeting is punctual, which can considerably limit the impact of the help provided. This lack of follow-up also forces the person in distress to repeat his or her story every time.

> We see the first signs of distress in the chat, we feel that the person is not well. The person is invited to redirect to Discord and take a ticket. (CM_AB3_F)

In addition, like any person in a care and help situation, emotional fatigue is a danger for all helpers, and in this case, helpers might also face "digital fatigue" (Collins-Pisano et al. 2021). The mental health concerns and the psychological distress of gamers can directly affect helpers. Their roles are also time-consuming. With the high volume of requests, they can feel overwhelmed and may put their mental health at risk and experience psychological and physical exhaustion.

> Some people have attachment issues. We must put limits, so that it remains healthy for the teams but also the ones in distress. (CM_AB3_F)

Many gamers then spontaneously or circumstantially take on the role of helper in order to support their peers. However, they may not have the skills to provide constructive assistance. In some cases, the advice provided may not be adequate, can be misinformation, or even be unwelcome (Kaplan et al. 2011; Li et al. 2015). Moreover, when two gamers with fragile mental health interact with each other, the positive effects of mutual aid can diminish or even become counterproductive. In the case of feelings of distress, sometimes related to suicide and self-harm, the pain and experiences shared by a gamer can create, awaken, or amplify this same feeling of distress in another gamer's life. Support related to peer help is no longer possible, and a third party's intervention becomes necessary to stop a negative spiral.

> It is sometimes the case that the person helping is very fragile themselves and helping someone else is a big burden. In the end, it is not necessarily beneficial for either. Sometimes, we even have to intervene with the person who tried to help, because they had put themselves in distress by doing so. (CM_AB3_F)

This kind of situation happens when high-volume communities cannot filter messages requiring immediate intervention, involve someone with intervention training, or help gamers in distress at late hours. Indeed, several support and peer support services are only active during the day and evening, leaving gamers in need unassisted at night.

As we have seen previously, the instinct of some gamers who witness a problem will be to redirect people in distress to external help, official suicide prevention services, and addiction assistance. This form of mutual aid is made available through messages pinned in Discord, including various links to specialized organizations. However, some will not want to seek help outside the safe space of the gaming community.

In addition, assessing the severity, and even the veracity, of particular distress messages can sometimes be challenging. Some victims may feel that they are not being heard or helped. There are several reasons why gamers in need can feel this. Sometimes they cannot carry through with the advice given, are not attentive, or do not even perceive that help is being offered. Li, Chen, and Popiel (2015) confirm that support is sometimes not perceived or felt. They distinguished two types of peer-to-peer support on Facebook: real support and perceived support. The actual support received does not systematically meet the need for support of the person targeted for support. Support can be information given, advice, or benevolent messages, but it can miss the mark or even contradict what the person actually needs, and therefore, they will not perceive this as support. However, perceived support is what is expected by the person suffering and what they deserve. For this, it requires involvement, follow-up care, and professionalism, which is not guaranteed in the context of video game peer help.

## Conclusion

In this paper, a portrait of peer support in gaming communities was drawn by directly questioning the people concerned. Many benefits have been raised regarding better mental health, starting with feeling part of a community, coming out of isolation, and opening communication channels in a safe space inhabited by fellow human beings. Simply playing, sharing a passion, and spending time on different gaming platforms and social media can positively contribute to good mental health.

We often hear about toxicity in video games, but the structures of the games can also encourage mutual aid relationships. Game features that promote stable, long-term social relationships ensure greater group cohesion. Unlike matchmaking which impersonalizes players, features like friend lists or long-term teams encourage recognition of others and empathy. In the same way, non-competition between members of the same group promotes a better context for social cohesion. For example, the competition between members' teams in LEAGUE OF LEGENDS (Riot, 2009) and the fact that not everyone has the same objectives at the same time harms social cohesion. Conversely, games where everyone has the same objectives and the same rewards, like GUILD WARS 2 (ArenaNet, 2012), promote mutual aid between players (Bonenfant et al., 2018).

By structuring the roles in play and then the social roles, the games promote, or not, a normalization of mutual aid within the game. Peer support between gamers is often held by online chats or other spaces of communication like Discord or Twitch. But the game structures such as guilds or long-term teams influence the way gamers will organize mutual aid by reproducing this social structure to respond to requests for help. Usually through mentoring, the response to this request for help can be expanded through peer help in mental health contexts.

During the COVID-19 pandemic, this normalization of mutual aid had concrete effects. Several informal organizations founded by gamers have emerged to assist gamers in distress during lockdowns. This peer help proved so effective that requests quickly exceeded the ability of stakeholders and moderators to respond to all gamers in need. Some gamers then spontaneously took over, demonstrating the empathy and solidarity of the community towards their neighbors. Many gamers said in interviews that they received invaluable help that made them feel better and avoid self-harm or even suicide.

Despite these positive attributes of mutual assistance between gamers, re-search participants raised many drawbacks: exhaustion of caregivers, insufficient help offered, night time slots without service, no follow-up with the ones in need, and inadequate or unprofessional responses from peers. Nevertheless, this research confirms the findings of Naslund et al. (2016a) that while the risk of misinformation and inappropriate comments exists, peer support on social media brings more benefits to the individual than harm. Peer help in a video game context is undoubtedly a crucial social safety net: interacting in-game and on community communication platforms, gamers all have the potential to become sentinels who can identify who is suffering and offer help to the extent of their means.

While these conclusions seem straightforward, they remain context specific since the participants are all Francophones living in Quebec who play certain types of games. It is impossible to generalize findings to the 3 billion gamers in the world. Differences are undoubtedly observable in other games, other lan-guage communities, or other regions of the world. We are well aware of the progressive and social democratic context of Quebec, where the state funds many social services. A social culture where helping others is normalized reflects this desire to help others.

However, this culture of mutual aid should not minimize the role of government in mental health. For this reason, the frontline social safety net offered by the gaming community should be further supported by the government by providing more funding to the second line, which is mental health professionals and non-profit organizations that can back up peer support by offering help at any time of the day, with necessary follow-up care over a long period, adequate responses, or even redirection to specialized medical services. In order to do so, the first step is to recognize the contribution of video games to the lives of many individuals and to destigmatize video game practice. By doing so, the transition from the first to the second line will be facilitated and we can confidently say that gaming saves lives.

## Annex: questions for the semistructured interviews

### Gamer Profile

- Can you tell me about the place of video games in your life?
- When did you start playing?
- What type(s) of practice have you had in your life? (single-player, online, for how long per day/week?)
- Who do you usually play with?
- Do you communicate with other gamers in the game? Or would you rather play alone?
- Do you participate in exchanges with other gamers outside of the game? (Twitch, Discord, Reddit, etc.)?
- Generally, do you consider yourself involved in the gamer's community? Do you feel a sense of belonging?

### Prosocial or Toxic Behaviors

- Generally, do you find that gamers are more benevolent or toxic? Can you explain your answer?

- What were the specifics in the context of the game? Have you ever witnessed situations where a gamer has helped another? Which?
- Have you ever helped a gamer in the circumstances?
- Or conversely, have you ever witnessed manifestations of toxicity?
- What form(s) did this toxicity take? Was it about the game? Or was it about the gamer's life?
- Have you ever been toxic to another gamer within a game? What were the circumstances?
- Are there games where behaviors are more benevolent? Or more toxic?
- How do you think behaviors could be encouraged Benevolent in video games?
- Conversely, how can toxic behavior be curbed?

### Peer Support Experience

- Have you ever witnessed situations where one gamer helped another in his or her life (played a moral support role)? Can you tell me about the circumstances?
- Have you ever helped a gamer in-game? If you feel like it, will you tell me the circumstances?
- Have you ever been helped by another gamer? If you feel like it, will you tell me the circumstances?
- Do you think these moral support situations are common in gaming communities?
- Do you think gamers can assume the role of"front line" by mental health? Is there a social safety net in the gamer's communities for distressed gamers?
- How could things be improved to help gamers who need it better?

### Repercussions

- What would you say to a non-gamer if you had to convince him/her of the benefits of playing video games?
- Conversely, are there any negative aspects to playing video games?
- What are the impacts on your life outside of the games? Positive? Negative?

## References

Ahmad, M. A., Huffaker, D., Wang, J., Treem, J., Kumar, D., Poole, M. S. & Srivastava, J. (2010). The Many Faces of Mentoring in an MMORPG. In 2010 *IEEE Second International Conference on Social Computing* (p. 270–275). IEEE.

Andalibi, N. & Flood M. K. (2021). Considerations in Designing Digital Peer Support for Mental Health: Interview Study Among Users of a Digital Support System (Buddy Project). *JMIR Mental Health*, 8(1).

Anderson, B. (1983), Imagined communities, Reflections on the origin and spread of nationalism, Verso.

Barr, M., Copeland-Steward A. (2021, May 6). Playing Video Games During the COVID-19 Pandemic and Effects on Players' Well-Being *Games and Culture*. 2022;17(1):122-139. https://doi.org/10.1177%2F15554120211017036

Bender, J. L., Jimenez-Marroquin, M. C., & Jadad, A. R. (2011). Seeking support on Facebook: a content analysis of breast cancer groups. *Journal of medical Internet Research*, 13(1), e16. https://doi.org/10.2196/jmir.1560

Bengtsson, T. T., Bom, L. H., Fynbo, L. (2021). Playing Apart Together: Young People's Online Gaming During the COVID-19 Lockdown. *YOUNG*, 29(4), 65–S80. https://doi.org/10.1177%2F11033088211032018

Berry, N., Lobban, F., Belousov, M., Emsley, R., Nenadic, G., & Bucci, S. (2017). #WhyWeTweetMH: Understanding Why People Use Twitter to Discuss Mental Health Problems. *Journal of Medical Internet Research*, 19(4), e107. https://doi.org/10.2196/jmir.6173

Bonenfant, M., Lafrance St-Martin, L.I., Prégent, F. & Crémier, L. (2018). Social systems and behavioral norms: the comparative case study of Guild Wars II and League of Legends. In Lakkaraju, Kiran, Sukthankar, Gita (Ed.). *Social Interaction in Virtual Worlds*, Cambridge University Press: 130–161.

Castronova, E. (2008). Exodus to the Virtual World: How Online Fun In Changing Reality, *Medienimpulse*, 49(1). https://doi.org/10.21243/mi-01-11-14

Chao, CM., Yu, TK. Internet Use and Adolescents' Physical and Mental Health: the Mediating Role of Self-consciousness and Peer Relationships. *Int J Ment Health Addiction* (2021). https://doi.org/10.1007/s11469-021-00631-x

Chou, W. Y., Hunt, Y., Folkers, A., & Augustson, E. (2011). Cancer survivorship in the age of YouTube and social media: a narrative analysis. *Journal of Medical Internet Research*, 13(1), e7. https://doi.org/10.2196/jmir.1569

Collins-Pisano, C., Velez Court, J., Johnson, M., Mois, G., Brooks, J., Myers, A., Muralidharan, A., Storm, M., Wright, M., Berger, N., Kasper, A., Fox, A., MacDonald, S., Schultze, S., & Fortuna, K. (2021). Core Competencies to Promote Consistency and Standardization of Best Practices for Digital Peer Support: Focus Group Study. *JMIR Mental Health*, 8(12). https://doi.org/10.2196/30221

Domahidi, E., Festl, R., Quandt, T. (2014). To dwell among gamers: Investigating the relationship between social online game use and gaming-related friendships, *Computers in Human Behavior*.

Fortuna, K. L., Solomon, P., & Rivera, J. (2022). An Update of Peer Support/Peer Provided Services Underlying Processes, Benefits, and Critical Ingredients. *The Psychiatric Quarterly*, 93(2), 571–586. https://doi.org/10.1007/s11126-022-09971-w

Fortuna, K. L., Myers, A. L., Ferron, J., Kadakia, A., Bianco, C., Bruce, M. L. & Bartels, S. J. (2021). Assessing a Digital Peer Support Self-Management Intervention for

Adults With Serious Mental Illness: Feasibility, Acceptability, and Preliminary Effectiveness. *Journal of Mental Health*.

Fortuna, K. L., Myers, A. L., Walsh, D., Walker, R., Mois, G., & Brooks, J. M. (2020a). Strategies to Increase Peer Support Specialists' Capacity to Use Digital Technology in the Era of COVID-19: Pre-Post Study. JMIR mental health, 7(7), e20429. https://doi.org/10.2196/20429

Fortuna, K. L., Naslund, J. A., LaCroix, J. M., Bianco, C. L., Brooks, J. M., Zisman-Ilani, Y., Muralidharan, A. & Deegan, P. (2020b). Digital Peer Support Mental Health Interventions for People With a Lived Experience of a Serious Mental Illness: Systematic Review. JMIR Mental Health, 7(4). https://pubmed.ncbi.nlm.nih.gov/32243256/

Fortuna, K. L., Venegas, M., Umucu, E., Mois, G., Walker, R. & Brooks, J. M. (2019). The Future of Peer Support in Digital Psychiatry: Promise, Progress, and Opportunities. *Current Treatment Options in Psychiatry*, 6, 221–231.

Frohlich, D. O., & Zmyslinski-Seelig, A. (2012). The presence of social support messages on YouTube videos about inflammatory bowel disease and ostomies. *Health communication*, 27(5), 421–428. https://doi.org/10.1080/10410236.2011.606524

Griffiths K. M. Reynolds J. Vassallo S. (2015). An Online, Moderated Peer-to-Peer Support Bulletin Board for Depression: User-Perceived Advantages and Disadvantages. *JMIR Mental Health*, 2(2), e14. 10.2196/mental.426626543919 https://mental.jmir.org/2015/2/e14/

Halbrook, Y., O'Donnell, A., Msetfi, R. (2019). When and how video games can be good: a review of the positive effects of video games on well-being. *Perspectives on Psychological Science*; 14 (6).

Homo Ludens. (2021). Usages et appropriations du jeu vidéo *Animal Crossing: New Horizons* en contexte de pandémie.

Johannes, N., Vuorre, M., & Przybylski, A. K. (2020, November 13). Video game play is positively correlated with well-being. https://doi.org/10.1098/rsos.202049

Kaplan K. Salzer M. S. Solomon P. Brusilovskiy E. Cousounis P. (2011). Internet peer support for individuals with psychiatric disabilities: A randomized controlled trial. *Social Science & Medicine*, 72(1), 54–62. https://doi.org/10.1016/j.socscimed.2010.09.03721112682

Karsenti, T. & Bugmann, J. (2018). Le e-sport, un nouveau « sport » numérique universitaire? *Revue internationale des technologies en pédagogie universitaire*, 15(1), 74–87.

Lenhart, A., Smith, A., Anderson, M., Duggan, M., & Perrin, A. (2015). Teens, technology, and friendships. *Pew Research Center*. Retrieved from http://www.pewinternet.org/2015/08/06/teens-technology-and-friendships/

Lewis, J.E, Trojovsky, M., Jameson, M. M. (2021). New Social Horizons: Anxiety, Isolation and Animal Crossing during the COVID-19 Pandemic. *Frontiers in Virtual Reality*. DOI: https://doi.org/10.3389/frvir.2021.627350

Li, X., W. Chen, and P. Popiel (2015). What happens on Facebook stays on Facebook? The implications of Facebook interaction for perceived, receiving, and giving social support. *Computers in Human Behavior*, 51, 106–113. https://doi.org/10.1016/j.chb.2015.04.066

Martončik M. et al. (2016). Do World of Warcraft (MMORPG) players experience less loneliness and social anxiety in online world (virtual environment) than in real world (offline)?, *Computers in Human Behavior*.

Merchant, R., Goldin, A., Manjanatha, D., Harter, C., Chandler, J., Lipp, A., Nguyen, T., Naslund, J. (2022). Opportunities to expand access to mental health services: A case for the role of online peer support communities, *The Psychiatric Quarterly*. DOI: DOI:10.1007/s11126-022-09974-7

Mertan, E., Croucher, L., Shafran, R., & Bennett, S. D. (2020). An investigation of the information provided to the parents of young people with mental health needs on an Internet forum. *Internet interventions*, *23*, 100353. https://doi.org/10.1016/j.invent.2020.100353

Nardi, B. (2006). Collaborative Play in World of Warcraft. In *2006 Fourth Latin American Web Congress* (p. 149–158). IEEE.

Naslund, J.A., Aschbrenner, K.A., Marsch, L.A., MacHugo, G.J., Bartels, S.J. (2018).Facebook for Supporting a Lifestyle Intervention for People with Major Depressive Disorder, Bipolar Disorder, and Schizophrenia: an Exploratory Study. *Psychiatr Q* 89, 81–94.

Naslund, J.A, Aschbrenner, K.A, Marsch, L. A., Bartels, S.J. (2016a). *The future of mental health care: peer-to-peer support and social media.* Epidemiology and Psychiatric Sciences, 25(2): 113–122.

Naslund, J. A., Aschbrenner, K. A., Marsch, L. A., & Bartels, S. J. (2016b). Feasibility and acceptability of Facebook for health promotion among people with serious mental illness. *Digital health*, 2, 2055207616654822. https://doi.org/10.1177/2055207616654822

Naslund, J.A., Aschbrenner, K.A, Grande, S. W., Elwyn, G. (2014). Naturally Occurring Peer Support through Social Media: The Experiences of Individuals with Severe Mental Illness Using YouTube, *PLoS*, 9(10). DOI: http://dx.doi.org/10.1371/journal.pone.0110171.

O'Leary, K., Schueller, S., Wobbrock, J., Pratt; W. (2018), Suddenly, we got to become therapists for each other: Designing Peer support Chats for Mental Health. *Proceedings of the 2018 CHI Conference.* http://dx.doi.org/10.1145/3173574.3173905

Pearce, C (2011). *Communities of Play, Emergent Cultures in Multiplayer Games and Virtual Worlds*. The MIT Press.

Rusk, F., Ståhl, M. & Silseth, K. (2020). Exploring peer mentoring and learning among experts and novices in online in-game interactions. *14th Proceedings of the European conference on games-based learning*, Brighton, 461–468.

Sangeorzan, I., Andriopoulou, P., Livanou, M. (2019). Exploring the experiences of people vlogging about severe mental illness on YouTube: An interpretative phenomenological analysis. *Journal of Affective Disorders*, 246(November), 422–428. 10.1016/j.jad.2018.12.11930599364

Schiano, D. et al., (2011), A new look at World of Warcraft's social landscape, *Proceedings of the 6th International Conference on Foundations of Digital Games – FDG '11*.

Simon, B., Boudreau, K. et Silverman, M. (2009). Two Players: Biography and 'Played Sociality' in EverQuest. *Game Studies*, 9(1).

Strand, M., Eng, L. S., Gammon, D. (2020). Combining online and offline peer support groups in community mental health care settings: A qualitative study of service users' experiences. *International Journal of Mental Health Systems*, 14(1), 39. 10.1186/s13033-020-00370-x32514303

Sundberg, M. (2018). Online gaming, loneliness, and friendships among adolescents and adults with ASD. *Computers in Human Behavior, pp. 79*, 105–110.

Taylor, T. L (2006). *Play Between Worlds: Exploring Online Game Culture.* The MIT Press.

Zhu, L. (2020). The psychology behind video games during COVID-19 pandemic: A case study of Animal Crossing: New Horizons. *Hum Behav & Emerg Tech.*, pp. 3, 157–159. https://doi.org/10.1002/hbe2.221

# On the Potential of Digital Games to Promote Healthy and Pro-Environmental Behavior

*Marco Rüth*

Environmental changes have been negatively affecting health worldwide. Particularly climate change is expected to have a range of negative impacts on the health of about 3.6 billion people, including higher rates of physical diseases and mental health issues (Khraishah et al., 2022; Palinkas & Wong, 2020; WHO, 2023). Thereby, climate change could aggravate the existing high prevalence of global health problems as well as other health-related crises due to, for instance, insufficient physical activity, pandemics, and a decrease in biodiversity (e.g., Hall et al., 2020; Marselle et al., 2021). Thus, healthy and pro-environmental behavior are interrelated and can influence each other, and it remains important to highlight this connection to make climate change and other environmental challenges more relevant to people (cf. Campbell et al., 2023; Maibach et al., 2010).

Different measures have been discussed to assess health risks, to prevent environmental damage, and to adapt to environmental changes (e.g., WHO, 2013, 2023). Still, while raising relevance, awareness, and knowledge have been important, a core issue is to convey and retain the urgency to act upon health and environmental changes and crises. In fact, a lack of mitigation of and adaption to climate change were among the most important short-term and long-term global risks, emphasizing that adaptation measures and behavior change are both important and urgent (WEF, 2023). However, more recent data from 2025 indicate that several environmental risks are still considered in the long-term, but less frequently in the short-term (WEF, 2025). Nevertheless, the need for adaptation and behavior change remains, and behavior change can be a powerful driver towards a more sustainable future (IPCC, 2023; Pathak et al., 2022). Hence, the promotion of healthy and pro-environmental behavior is a key global challenge.

Healthy behavior supports in reaching or maintaining health as the "state of complete physical, mental, and social well-being" (WHO, 2021, p. 1) and includes sufficient physical activity, a balanced diet as well as enjoyable and stress-relieving activities. Pro-environmental behavior refers to behavior that "consciously protects the environment and improves its sustainability" (Tian & Liu, 2022, p. 2) and includes saving natural resources, preventing environmental issues, and pursuing a sustainable lifestyle. One way to foster healthy and pro-environmental behavior can be using digital games, i.e., digital interactive media that contain game elements, such as goals, challenges, or feedback (cf. Rüth, 2022).

Digital games have been used to increase engagement in healthy and pro-environmental behavior and can support the prevention, treatment, and rehabilitation of physical and mental health conditions (Colder Carras et al., 2018). According to systematic literature reviews, digital games have been frequently used in health contexts regarding physical activity, rehabilitation, and quality of life (e.g., Boyle et al., 2016; Connolly et al., 2012). For instance, some uses of digital commercial games and serious games – games with the primary aim to improve specific outcomes such as health outcomes and with the secondary aim to entertain – were found to result in similar or better health and quality of life compared to traditional therapy and rehabilitation approaches (e.g., Rüth et al., 2023; Zayeni et al., 2020). Playing and watching digital games can also support in experiencing and conveying mental health topics (e.g., Kasdorf, 2023; Rüth et al., 2025). Moreover, digital games that focus on processes and impacts of climate change and possible actions can provide meaningful and immersive experiences that foster the engagement of people and make related topics more tangible (e.g., Koroleva & Novak, 2020; op de Beke et al., 2024; Wu & Lee, 2015). Further, people seem to engage more in climate action when they play both digital games generally and digital games that include content about global warming specifically (Carman et al., 2024). Such findings are promising, yet it is crucial to put a stronger emphasis on the role of environmental factors in peoples' physical and mental health, also regarding health and environmental crises (e.g., Dadaczynski et al., 2023; Kermavnar et al., 2023; Maibach et al., 2010). Against this background, I scrutinize why and how using digital games can effectively promote healthy and pro-environmental behavior.

First, I outline why digital games can be used to promote healthy and pro-environmental behavior. Second, I consider empirical evidence on effects of digital games on healthy and pro-environmental behavior. Third, I delineate avenues for the design of and research on digital games that aim to promote healthy and pro-environmental behavior.

## Digital games as tools to promote healthy and pro-environmental behavior

There are several reasons why digital games can be effective at fostering healthy and pro-environmental behavior. In what follows, these reasons are clustered in terms of characteristics of digital games, theoretical considerations, and reasons related to healthy and pro-environmental behavior.

## Characteristics of digital games and behavior change

Several characteristics of digital games may qualify them as effective tools for behavior change.

First, digital games are popular interactive media that can reach large audiences and that can go beyond information and knowledge transmission. In fact, digital games are used by more than three billion people worldwide, with more people using mobile games (83%) than PC games (26%) and console games (18%) (Newzoo, 2025). So, digital games can unfold their effects in home or mobile environments as well as in educational, health, and professional contexts (e.g., Damaševičius et al., 2023; Hammady & Arnab, 2022; Rüth & Kaspar, 2020, 2021a). For instance, it was found that physical activity or healthy eating habits can be fostered by means of self-developed or commercial digital games – for instance, Nintendo's WII SPORTS or WII FIT games – that offer rewards, challenges, and feedback mechanisms (e.g., Hammady & Arnab, 2022; Rüth et al., 2023).

Second, digital games can provide suitable environments for active learning, safe environments for experimentation of solutions for complex problems, and scalable environments to address and connect large audiences (Creutzig & Kapmeier, 2020). More specifically, games that enable solving complex problems and provide challenging experiences can be beneficial for behavior change (Hammady & Arnab, 2022). For instance, digital games such as ANNO 2070, CIVILIZATION VI: GATHERING STORM, PLAGUE INC: EVOLVED, and STOP DISASTERS allow to experience dynamics, decisions, and consequences with respect to city management, pandemics, and environmental disasters (e.g., Fernández Galeote & Hamari, 2021; Gampell & Gaillard, 2016; Kelly, 2020).

Third, looking at behavior change as a learning process, game-based learning includes several aspects that can foster affective, behavioral, cognitive, and social/cultural engagement (Plass et al., 2020). These aspects can also be understood in terms of game elements and learning elements that can foster motivation (Proulx et al., 2017). More specifically, digital games can provide rewards if intended behavior is performed or contain predefined sequences to guide users toward intended behavior and away from unintended behavior (Hammady & Arnab, 2022). For instance, the scenario *Eden Burning* in the digital game ANNO 1800 includes the so-called eco balance, i.e., information about water quality, soil quality, and air quality (Ubisoft, 2021). These environmental metrics decrease due to, for instance, pesticide use or air pollution via factories, and increase due to, for instance, water purification plants or forestation.

To sum up, these characteristics and examples illustrate the potential of digital games for changing healthy and pro-environmental behavior. Still, the way in which games represent and implement health and environmental topics is also subject to debate and criticism (e.g., Damaševičius et al., 2023; op de Beke et al., 2024). In the following, I discuss how theoretical considerations can support progress toward effective digital games for behavior change.

## Theoretical considerations on digital games and behavior change

Why digital games can support behavior change can also be understood in terms of numerous theoretical frameworks (Krath et al., 2021). Frequently used frameworks regarding games as well as healthy and pro-environmental behavior change include the theory of planned behavior, social cognitive theory, and self-determination theory (e.g., Beauchamp et al., 2019; Hammady & Arnab, 2022; Ntoumanis et al., 2021; Yuriev et al., 2020).

The theory of planned behavior states that behavior can be predicted by intention toward the behavior (behavioral intention), by attitude toward the behavior (attitude), by considerations on the extent to which the behavior is expected from others (subjective norm), and by the perceived ability to perform the behavior (perceived behavioral control) (Ajzen, 2020). According to meta-analytic results, using digital serious games for health has small effects on some behavioral determinants, namely attitudes, the belief in one's capability to perform actions (self-efficacy, a construct related to perceived behavioral control), and behavioral intention (DeSmet et al., 2014). Moreover, a systematic review shows that using digital serious games and gamified apps increased attitudes or self-efficacy and fostered pro-environmental behavior (Boncu et al., 2022). The theory of planned behavior may provide some explanatory value, yet it was also found that a gamified app can directly promote pro-environmental behavior without changing attitudes or beliefs (Boncu et al., 2023).

Social cognitive theory also aims to explain what motivates human behavior by considering the interplay of personal (e.g., goals and self-efficacy), behavioral (e.g., choice and effort), and environmental factors (e.g., social models and feedback) (Schunk & DiBenedetto, 2020). In general, digital games can address several of these factors, for instance, by providing opportunities for observational learning and learning from others via role models and multiplayer modes (Krath et al., 2021; Rüth & Kaspar, 2020). More specifically, digital serious and commercial games were found to increase adolescents' and adults' self-efficacy regarding physical activity and pro-environmental behavior (Fox et al., 2020; Staiano et al., 2017). Further, it was found that self-efficacy is higher after interactive play than after watching gameplay videos (Peng, 2008; Lee, 2015), so playing rather than watching digital games could increase self-efficacy and foster behavior change.

According to self-determination theory, reasons for why digital games can be engaging include their potential to satisfy the basic psychological needs for autonomy, competence, and relatedness (e.g., Cheek et al., 2015; Krath et al., 2021; Proulx et al., 2017). More specifically, relevant goals and own choices can foster a sense of ownership (need for autonomy), clear goals and feedback can support a feeling of success (need for competence), and collaboration and teams can create a sense of belonging (need for relatedness). For instance, it was found that the need for competence can be addressed by providing badges for completing goals or levels, leaderboards with information about one's performance in relation to others, and performance graphs that inform about one's own change in performance (Sailer et al., 2017). Notably, it has been discussed to expand the set of basic psychological needs, for instance, by considering the need for novel experiences (Vansteenkiste et al., 2020).

Taken together, digital games can promote healthy and pro-environmental behavior since they address key constructs delineated in theories on motivation and behavior change. Several constructs contained in these theories are related (e.g., perceived behavioral control, self-efficacy, and need for competence), and these and other theories can be adapted to research and practice contexts.

## Digital games and healthy and pro-environmental behavior

There are also more specific reasons for why digital games can effectively promote healthy and pro-environmental behavior.

First, digital games can provide a sense of agency with engaging and immersive experiences that elicit strong cognitive, affective, and behavioral engagement and responses in the context of climate change – examples include Eco, Keep Cool, World Rescue, and Tree (e.g., Fernández Galeote et al., 2021; Fernández Galeote & Hamari, 2021; Spangenberger et al., 2024; Wu & Lee, 2015). Still, agency and actions in virtual environments may also hamper the level of engagement in the real world, for instance, due to the impression that environmental problems have already been solved in the virtual world (cf. Fletcher, 2017). So, it is important to distinguish between the motivation to play games as well as engagement and actions within games, on the one hand, and engagement, behavior, and effects in the real world, on the other.

Second, digital games can make use of persuasive mechanisms, such as rewards, self-monitoring, personalization, and cooperation or competition. For instance, games using persuasive mechanisms were found to have positive effects on disease management, nutrition, physical activity, environmental sustainability, and environmental citizenship (Georgiou et al., 2023; Ndulue & Orji, 2022). More specifically, behavior change in these contexts has been facilitated via competition or cooperation in the form of leaderboards and challenges as well as self-monitoring and reduction in the form of progress bars and reduced task complexity (Ndulue & Orji, 2022). So, digital games may affect healthy and pro-environmental behavior via a range of persuasive mechanisms.

Third, digital games can provide social environments and experiences that are also important for learning, changing, and maintaining healthy and pro-environmental behavior (e.g., Greipl et al., 2020; Ndulue & Orji, 2022; Rüth & Kaspar, 2021a).

For instance, interviews with players who had played the game Eco for two to four weeks show that players see cooperation as key in the game due to its complexity, limited resources, and synergy effects through task sharing (Fjællingsdal & Klöckner, 2019). Further, playing or discussing together with others can allow players to receive or offer social support, to exchange perspectives, and to reflect on their behavior and even change it (cf. Rüth & Kaspar, 2021a, 2021b). However, a systematic review indicates that social aspects are among the least frequently used persuasive mechanisms in digital games that target healthy and pro-environmental behavior (Ndulue & Orji, 2022). Nevertheless, digital games can bring people together and thereby promote healthy and pro-environmental behavior.

Overall, this non-exhaustive list of reasons illustrates why digital games can be effective tools to promote healthy and pro-environmental behavior. Next, I focus on studies that examined how digital games foster specific types of healthy and pro-environmental behavior.

## On the potential of digital games to promote healthy behavior

Several studies have shown that digital games can promote healthy behavior. For instance, a meta-analysis investigated how digital serious games affect healthy lifestyles, including diet and physical activity, health responsibility and maintenance, social behavior, and mental health promotion (DeSmet et al., 2014). The analysis revealed small effects of digital serious games on health behavior based on 21 studies in the short term, yet no significant effect on health behavior based on ten studies in the long term. Nevertheless, there were small significant effects on clinical outcomes such as weight in the short and long term. The largest positive effects were found for smoking prevention and cessation, HIV-protective behavior, and nutritional behavior. While some of the studies evaluated interactive multimedia applications with rather few game elements, I shortly present two studies of the meta-analysis that used digital games.

In the first study, third-grade students completed a nutrition course in four weeks either using five digital games or multimedia slides (Yien et al., 2011). The digital games were about different topics, including food types, healthy eating habits, and relations between nutrition, health, and the environment. Students who played the games performed better in a knowledge test about nutrition and reported better eating and drinking habits after the course compared to the control group. While this study only compared two classes with 33 students each, these results indicate how using digital games about nutrition in primary school can positively affect the health of children. The second study showed that using two digital games can foster the nutritional behavior of children aged 10 to 12 outside of a school context, compared to using an internet-based learning experience that included game elements (Baranowski et al., 2011). The digital games were aimed at changing nutritional behavior and physical activity to lower the risk of obesity and type 2 diabetes. The games were based on social cognitive theory, self-determination theory, and persuasion theories, and offered several hours of gameplay. Eventually, children who played the games reported more intake of vegetables and fruits, but the physical activity did not increase based on accelerometry. So, these examples illustrate that using digital games can positively affect healthy behavior regarding nutrition.

Other studies have shown that using digital games can positively affect physical activity. For instance, a meta-analysis based on 19 longitudinal studies found moderate positive effects of a repeated use of exergames – games that require physical activity to be played – on overall physical activity (Moller et al., 2023). The overall methodological quality of the included studies was rather low due to, inter alia, lack of blinding. Here, I focus on the study with the highest quality ratings that evaluated how the weekly use of exergames affected the energy expenditure of 81 students in fourth grade during their school day (Gao et al., 2019). A fitness room was equipped with several consoles and commercial exergames, inter alia, JUST DANCE and WII FIT, that could be played in groups of up to four children, supervised by a physical education teacher. The students in the control group continued their regular physical activities, including the regular weekly physical education class. The main finding of this study was that the daily caloric expenditure increased in the intervention group and decreased in the control group. Complementary to these results, a systematic review shows that the use of commercial exergames in unsupervised home environments can also support adults in need of physical rehabilitation (Rüth et al., 2023). Of the 20 studies included in this review, 12 reported similar or higher effects of using exergames on physical health compared to, inter alia, receiving physical activity advice, continuing usual activities, and usual rehabilitation care. Additionally, 15 studies also examined quality of life, nine of which reported similar or higher effects of exergaming compared to, inter alia, tailored exercises, usual activities, and conventional exercises or therapy. So, exergames can promote physical and mental health in different audiences and contexts.

Promoting healthy behavior also means ceasing unhealthy behavior. For instance, a systematic review on using digital serious games for smoking prevention and cessation found that people stopped smoking in four of seven studies (Derksen et al., 2020). The only study that was assessed to be of good methodological quality was a three-group randomized trial that evaluated a health-related intervention based on social cognitive theory, the theory of planned behavior, and self-determination theory (An et al., 2013). The study included people who lived in the USA, were aged between 18 and 30, and had smoked in the previous 30 days. It was found that a significantly larger number of the 441 participants in the health-related intervention group achieved a 30-day abstinence from smoking after three months compared to the 446 participants in the control group who completed a six-week program on general lifestyle topics (23% vs. 11%). In the third group that also included peer coaching, even more participants achieved a significantly higher 30-day abstinence from smoking (31%). The weekly health-related intervention was targeted at behavior change and consisted of five steps: 1) reporting health behavior, 2) receiving tailored motivational messages, 3) receiving tailored goal-setting messages and social support, 4) receiving strategy messages, and 5) a summary of the current and past week. More specifically, the health-related intervention was a gamified website including weekly interactive goal setting, an avatar who encouraged participants to change their behavior, and a progress bar that monitored the behavior. So, this intervention included some game elements, namely avatar creation, storytelling, a theme, and social formation (Derksen et al., 2020). Overall, the study by An et al. (2013) illustrates that a gamified health-related intervention can effectively promote healthy behavior by ceasing unhealthy behavior.

Taken together, several studies showed that digital games and gamified applications can promote healthy behavior and improve health-related outcomes.

## On the potential of digital games to promote pro-environmental behavior

Whether digital games can promote pro-environmental behavior has also been examined by several studies. A systematic review on using digital games for pro-environmental knowledge, attitude, and behavior identified 14 studies on pro-environmental behavior change (Boncu et al., 2022). Overall, the results on behavior change were mixed, based on small samples, and often non-significant or only short-term. Five studies used digital serious games and nine studies used gamified apps to address mainly energy consumption, but also water consumption, food consumption, and mobility. For instance, regarding energy consumption, a gamified app was used that provided individual feedback on change in electricity use, learning opportunities to gain action-related knowledge (i.e., tips on electricity saving), and rewards (e.g., points when more people of households participated in the challenge) (Wemyss et al., 2019). Twenty-one households used the app for a competition between households, a further 21 households used the app for a collaboration within households, and another 40 households were in the control group. It was found that the competitive households and the collaborative households saved more energy than the 40 households in the control group. Overall, the gamified app allowed users to reduce energy consumption while participating in the challenges during the intervention, but one year later there was no difference in energy consumption. Still, this study indicates how cooperative or competitive modes in gamified environments can improve pro-environmental behavior.

Another systematic review on using gamification in the context of climate change investigated how game elements are related to cognitive, affective, and behavioral engagement as well as to game experience (Fernández Galeote et al., 2021). Of the 35 studies included in this review that reported behavioral engagement, 21 reported outcomes that referred to in-game behavior. Still, eight outcomes were related to individual behavior such as decrease in carbon footprint, and two outcomes referred to transfer into community decision-making. Of the 12 studies that were rated to be of high or medium methodological quality, eight reported positive qualitative or descriptive results and three reported positive quantitative findings. Additionally, two studies reported mixed qualitative or quantitative results. The most frequently used game elements regarding behavioral outcomes were about achievement and progression (e.g., challenges, levels, and feedback) and social aspects (e.g., cooperation or collaboration, competition, and customization), while frequent topics included droughts, floods, and high or rising temperatures.

For instance, in a study by Onencan and van de Walle (2018), there were seven teams of five policymakers, each of which played a game that aimed to increase situation awareness and familiarity with climate change risks. The serious game was about drought as a disaster due to climate change and included elements that motivate cooperation, such as shared goals, complementary information and roles, and rewards for joint actions compared to individual actions. The policymakers played six rounds of the game in the presence of three facilitators. Based on subjective ratings, objective performance, and in-game measurements, the situation awareness of the policymakers was higher after playing the game compared to before playing the game. However, situation awareness only translated into policy actions when policymakers had a high (vs. low) familiarity with climate change risks. The authors of the study discuss that the facilitators may have played an important role in increasing the familiarity of later participants by means of sharing experiences and stories based on past game sessions of earlier participants. Overall, the study illustrates how a game designed for decision-makers can increase their situation awareness and that additional facilitation and discussion regarding the game may foster behavior change.

More recently, an experimental study investigated the effects of playing a digital game in single player mode on pro-environmental intentions and behavior (Fernández Galeote et al., 2023). The game was self-paced and story-based, so that each participant received the same information about climate change. Notably, the game also contained minigames and framed climate change as a wellbeing issue, connecting healthy and pro-environmental behavior. In a nutshell, the game was about different future scenarios, causes and effects related to climate change, and possible actions. Participants were assigned to one of three groups to compare the effects of playing the game using a computer versus using a virtual reality device versus using a digital document with the same information. Subsequently, participants were shown six types of actions related to climate change and the option to not act. Pro-environmental behavior was examined ten days later by asking participants whether they had engaged in their intended actions. Of the 105 participants, 102 were willing to engage and 42 answered the follow-up questionnaire on pro-environmental behavior. It was found that the intervention inspired most respondents to engage in pro-environmental behavior (81%). Eventually, about half of the respondents engaged in pro-environmental behavior (57%), some still intended to do so (29%), and others have not done so or forgotten about it (14%). These and other effects were similar across the three groups, maybe because the groups were also quite similar regarding a rather text-intensive game (game conditions) and a text enhanced by narrative and visual features (control condition). Still, this study indicates that using digital games that consider relations between health and the environment can promote actual pro-environmental behavior.

In sum, these studies illustrate that digital games and gamified applications can foster pro-environmental behavior in various ways among different audiences.

## How could digital games promote healthy and pro-environmental behavior?

The last sections focused on potentials of digital games and thus on studies that show how games can promote healthy and pro-environmental behavior. Some studies reported small effects or non-significant results and there may be publication bias due to unpublished data. Nevertheless, the reviewed results suggest that game-based approaches can be seen as a complementary or alternative way of promoting healthy and pro-environmental behavior in the general population. Still, it seems to be less common to (explicitly) consider relations between health and environmental issues as well as healthy and pro-environmental behavior. Thus, in this section I first outline possible interrelations between digital games, healthy behavior, and pro-environmental behavior. Then, I discuss some recommendations for the design of games with the aim to promote healthy and pro-environmental behavior.

### Interrelations between digital games and healthy and pro-environmental behavior

Several interrelations between digital games, healthy behavior, and pro-environmental behavior are conceivable and depicted in Figure 1. The three circles in Figure 1 represent digital games, healthy behavior, and pro-environmental behavior, which can be understood in terms of the definitions provided in the introduction to this chapter. Additionally, the overlap of the three circles results in four intersections: (1) games for healthy behavior; (2) games for pro-environmental behavior; (3) relations between healthy and pro-environ-mental behavior; and (4) games for healthy and pro-environmental behavior. While mainly the first three approaches (1–3) have been outlined in the last sections, the combined approach (4) is discussed in the following. Taken together, these intersections can be considered when designing or evaluating games for healthy or pro-environmental behavior. In practice, games for healthy behavior and games for pro-environmental behavior may also be used subsequently to emphasize the relations between both behaviors. To enhance these approaches, effective games for healthy and pro-environmental behavior as well as discussions on how to design such games are needed.

*Figure 1: A conceptual framework for the design and evaluation of digital games with the aim to address healthy and pro-environmental behavior. The intersections show possible interrelations between digital games, healthy behavior, and pro-environmental behavior, including (1) games for healthy behavior, (2) games for pro-environmental behavior, (3) relations between healthy and pro-environmental behavior, and (4) games for healthy and pro-environmental behavior.*

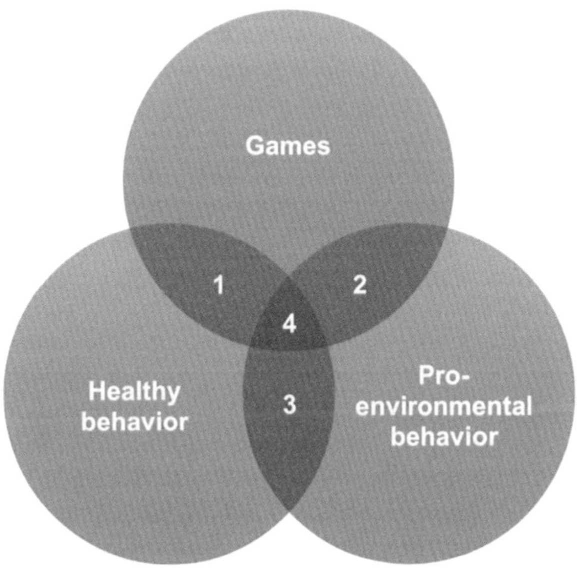

## Toward digital games for healthy and pro-environmental behavior

There is no simple or final answer on how to design digital games for healthy and pro-environmental behavior, which, however, has been discussed in several works (e.g., Cheek et al., 2015; Fizek et al., 2023; Gerber et al., 2021; Kuipers et al., 2017; Vervoort et al., 2022). Nevertheless, good practices regarding the design of games and gamified approaches have not been followed in several projects (e.g., de Salas et al., 2022). Here, I focus on how the design and use of games can benefit from considering theories and frameworks, empirical evidence, and further considerations related to behavior change.

## How theories and frameworks can inform the design of digital games

Theories can support the planning, design, implementation, and evaluation of behavior change games (cf. Willmott & Rundle-Thiele, 2021). Accordingly, several behavioral theories have been used to inform the design and use of games and gamified interventions for behavior change (e.g., de Salas et al., 2022; Hammady & Arnab, 2022).

As described at the beginning of this chapter, the theory of planned behavior, social cognitive theory, and self-determination theory as well as other theories may support in explaining why using digital games can change behavior (cf. Krath et al., 2021). Complementary to using theories, the potential of games to affect behavior change could be examined or increased by using specific frameworks such as for pro-environmental behavior (e.g., Ouariachi et al., 2019; Razali et al., 2022; White et al., 2019). For instance, a framework consisting of 15 game elements can be used to assess the cognitive, emotional, and behavioral engagement of games aimed at climate change behavior (Ouariachi et al., 2019, 2020). Other frameworks emphasize that potentials of games such as behavior change can unfold if key game elements are considered and that limits of games such as overstimulation may appear given too many or unsuitable game elements (Greipl et al., 2020; Rüth & Kaspar, 2021a).

Game design can also be informed by more general frameworks that highlight key elements for research and development projects, including goal setting and attainment, decision-making, and the consideration of different stakeholders, such as the general public, companies, non-governmental organizations, or politicians (cf. Rüth & Kaspar, 2017). More specifically, decision-making regarding the design and use of digital games should be justified and communicated more comprehensively, which is not yet always the case (e.g., de Salas et al., 2022).

So, there are multiple ways in which theories and frameworks can support the design and use of games.

## How empirical evidence can inform the design of digital games

Available evidence can be considered to identify potentials and limits of using games for healthy and pro-environmental behavior change (e.g., Boncu et al., 2022; Damaševičius et al., 2023; van Valkengoed & Steg, 2019). More specifically, digital games can build on strategies that have been used for years, for instance, narratives and framing to create suitable counter-narratives in health contexts such as smoking cessation (e.g., Malone & Proctor, 2022; cf. Rüth, 2025). Further, digital games can convey a constructive and solution-oriented perspective and make climate change adaptation and possible actions more tangible (cf. Fernández Galeote et al., 2023). Such actions can be aimed at the prevention of driving forces, hazard management, environmental improvements, protection of exposure, or correction of effects regarding climate change (WHO, 2013).

Key inhibitors of behavior change can also play an important role and include limited cognition, engagement in ineffective (low-cost) or compensatory behavior (rebound effect), and the preference for proximal (vs. distant) rewards (cf. Gifford, 2011). For instance, the health benefits of smoking cessation or the environmental benefits of using public transport may only become visible in the longer term. In this regard, it was found that one important factor for reaching goals with distant rewards is a high level of self-control, which was also found to play a role in pro-environmental behavior (Wyss et al., 2022). Moreover, challenges that people have not yet experienced and are related to distant goals can be made more proximal by means of game design. For instance, a gamified platform about flooding, water saving, water efficiency, and water reuse was found to motivate people to prepare for such circumstances (Koroleva & Novak, 2020). The core feature of the platform was a dashboard, and users stated that they were motivated by receiving points for reading articles and badges as achievements for reaching certain scores. The users also stated that social comparisons were motivating, for instance, since seeing points from other community members enabled them to see how well they do in comparison to others and to learn where they can help their community to prevent floods.

The findings of Koroleva and Novak (2020) also indicate that the motivational effect of gamification elements may vary between users with different characteristics or preferences. In this regard, the results of the meta-analysis of DeSmet et al. (2014) also suggest that tailoring games to socio-demographic information (e.g., age and gender) or behavior change needs (e.g., level of knowledge or lifestyle adoption) can effectively foster behavioral determinants and healthy behavior. Relatedly, one may also focus on specific target groups, such as on the nutrition-related behavior of younger adults who are particularly engaged in using online games (Micallef et al., 2022).

Taken together, these examples underline that game design can be informed by evidence related to the topic, the targeted behavior, and the target group.

## Further considerations on the design of digital games

Further considerations regarding the design of digital games include whether new games are needed or if modified or adapted versions of games can also effectively address healthy and pro-environmental behavior. In both cases, there are numerous game elements and persuasive mechanisms to choose from when it comes to designing and modifying games for behavior change (e.g., Fernández Galeote & Hamari, 2021; Georgiou et al., 2023). Relatedly, one could focus on designing games about topics regarding pro-environmental behavior that have been underrepresented in games about climate change (Fernández Galeote et al., 2021). Additionally, insights on how to effectively convey information about climate change or promote physical activity could facilitate the design and use of behavior change games (e.g., Campbell et al., 2023; de Meyer et al., 2020).

Since the main goal of the game is behavior change, it also remains important to outweigh how game elements and persuasive mechanisms foster engagement in the virtual and real world. Of course, games are designed to be appealing and entertaining, and game elements are commonly used to keep people playing. However, the goal of behavior change games should rather be to facilitate behavior change than to motivate to play or master the game (unless these goals largely overlap). Thus, connections to (behavior in) the real world are important for behavior change games to be effective. These connections could be strengthened by, for instance, increasing transfer effects of digital games or by using specific game elements in gamified contexts. In fact, numerous works have been discussing transfer effects of games for health (e.g., Baranowski et al., 2008, 2014; Kuipers et al., 2017). Moreover, most interventions using game elements for behavior change related to climate change were rather short and not facilitated (Fernández Galeote et al., 2021). In this regard, facilitators may support the transition from situation awareness to action and policymaking (Onencan & van de Walle, 2018).

Taken together, theories, evidence, and further considerations can facilitate the design and use of digital games to promote healthy and pro-environmental behavior.

## Future research on digital games for healthy and pro-environmental behavior

Future research on how games foster healthy and pro-environmental behavior can also be looked at in terms of theories, evidence, and further considerations related to behavior change.

First, regarding theories, it yet remains unclear whether the incorporation of theories results in more effective interventions aimed at health-related behavior change (Willmott & Rundle-Thiele, 2021). To assess this hypothesis, more works should include and report the theory for behavior change used in their studies in a consistent way. To support practical efforts, it remains important to highlight why, when, and how the use of theories could benefit behavior change. Thereby, the complexity of the targeted behaviors and the extent to which theories can address this complexity should be discussed. In this regard, a more thorough consideration of situational and practical aspects could facilitate the transfer from theoretical considerations to practical recommendations.

Second, more high-quality evidence is needed on the effectiveness of games for healthy and pro-environmental behavior for different audiences, in different contexts, and by means of different study designs and measurements (e.g., Lange, 2023; Lange & Dewitte, 2019; Rüth & Kaspar, 2021a). So, evaluating the effects of games remains important and should be based on suitable approaches (e.g., All et al., 2021; Mayer et al., 2014; Rüth, 2017). For instance, a thorough examination of behavior change may require several measurements at pre-game (e.g., status quo and moderators), in-game (e.g., events and changes throughout the game), and post-game (e.g., short-term and long-term effects). Additionally, the audiences and contexts in which games are played should be considered and reported to compare the effects of playing digital games with other approaches.

Third, healthy and pro-environmental behavior can be changed and investigated in many contexts. In this regard, touchpoints include events about game design and development such as game jams as well as several forms of citizen science and public engagement, including contributions to non-governmental organizations (e.g., Meriläinen, 2020; Partelow et al., 2020; Speelman et al., 2023). Further, future research could examine healthy and pro-environmental behavior as an interplay of bottom-up processes (e.g., individual actions or barriers) and top-down processes (e.g., governmental incentives or restrictions).

Overall, future efforts in research and development can make games more valuable and effective tools for encouraging healthy and pro-environmental behavior.

## Conclusion

Some studies have already shown how digital games and gamified apps can effectively promote healthy and pro-environmental behavior. However, several studies were not of high methodological quality according to systematic reviews, warranting future research. In this regard, I emphasized how digital games, healthy behavior, and pro-environmental behavior are interrelated, and that considering these interrelations could be a promising approach toward effective behavior change. Future efforts are also needed toward the design and use of digital games for audiences and about topics that have not yet been addressed. I delineated how such efforts can be supported by considering theories and frameworks, empirical evidence, and further considerations about the effective promotion of healthy and pro-environmental behavior. Finally, financing and disseminating effective games remains important to facilitate access to their potential effects. Overall, digital games have a potential to effectively foster healthy and pro-environmental behavior that has not yet been fully exploited.

## References

All, A., Castellar, E. N. P., & Van Looy, J. (2021). Digital game-based learning effectiveness assessment: Reflections on study design. *Computers & Education, 167*, 104160. https://doi.org/10.1016/j.compedu.2021.104160

An, L. C., Demers, M. R., Kirch, M. A., Considine-Dunn, S., Nair, V., Dasgupta, K., Narisetti, N., Resnicow, K., & Ahluwalia, J. (2013). A randomized trial of an avatar-hosted multiple behavior change intervention for young adult smokers. *Journal of the National Cancer Institute Monographs, 2013*, 209–215. https://doi.org/10.1093/jncimonographs/lgt021

Baranowski, T., Buday, R., Thompson, D. I., & Baranowski, J. (2008). Playing for real: video games and stories for health-related behavior change. *American Journal of Preventive Medicine, 34*, 74–82. https://doi.org/10.1016/j.amepre.2007.09.027

Baranowski, T., Baranowski, J., Thompson, D., Buday, R., Jago, R., Griffith, M. J., Islam, N., Nguyen, N., & Watson, K. B. (2011). Video game play, child diet, and physical activity behavior change: A randomized clinical trial. *American Journal of Preventive Medicine, 40*, 33–38. https://doi.org/10.1016/j.amepre.2010.09.029

Baranowski, M. T., Fiellin, P. L. E., Gay, G., & Thompson, D. I. (2014). Using what's learned in the game for use in real life. *Games For Health: Research, Development, and Clinical Applications, 3*, 6–9. https://doi.org/10.1089/g4h.2014.1715

Beauchamp, M. R., Crawford, K. L., & Jackson, B. (2019). Social cognitive theory and physical activity: Mechanisms of behavior change, critique, and legacy. *Psychology of Sport and Exercise, 42*, 110–117. https://doi.org/10.1016/j.psychsport.2018.11.009

Boncu, Ș., Candel, O. S., & Popa, N. L. (2022). Gameful green: a systematic review on the use of serious computer games and gamified mobile apps to foster pro-environmental information, attitudes and behaviors. *Sustainability, 14*, 10400. https://doi.org/10.3390/su141610400

Boncu, Ș., Candel, O. S., Prundeanu, O., & Popa, N. L. (2023). Growing a digital iceberg for a polar bear: effects of a gamified mobile app on university students' pro-environmental behaviours. *International Journal of Sustainability in Higher Education*. https://doi.org/10.1108/IJSHE-03-2023-0092

Boyle, E. A., Hainey, T., Connolly, T. M., Gray, G., Earp, J., Ott, M., Lim, T., Ninaus, M., Ribeiro, C., & Pereira, J. (2016). An update to the systematic literature review of empirical evidence of the impacts and outcomes of computer games and serious games. *Computers & Education, 94*, 178–192. https://doi.org/10.1016/j.compedu.2015.11.003

Campbell, E., Uppalapati, S. S., Kotcher, J., & Maibach, E. (2023). Communication research to improve engagement with climate change and human health: A review. *Frontiers in Public Health, 10*, 1086858. https://doi.org/10.3389/fpubh.2022.1086858

Carman, J. P., Psaros, M., Rosenthal, S. A., Marlon, J., Verner, M., Lee, S., … & Leiserowitz, A. (2024). Geeks versus climate change: understanding American video gamers' engagement with global warming. *Climatic Change, 177*, 85. https://doi.org/10.1007/s10584-024-03747-w

Cheek, C., Fleming, T., Lucassen, M. F., Bridgman, H., Stasiak, K., Shepherd, M., & Orpin, P. (2015). Integrating health behavior theory and design elements in serious games. *JMIR Mental Health, 2*, e4133. https://doi.org/10.2196/mental.4133

Colder Carras, M., Van Rooij, A. J., Spruijt-Metz, D., Kvedar, J., Griffiths, M. D., Carabas, Y., & Labrique, A. (2018). Commercial video games as therapy: A new research agenda to unlock the potential of a global pastime. *Frontiers in Psychiatry, 8*, 300. https://doi.org/10.3389/fpsyt.2017.00300

Connolly, T. M., Boyle, E. A., MacArthur, E., Hainey, T., & Boyle, J. M. (2012). A systematic literature review of empirical evidence on computer games and serious games. *Computers & Education, 59*, 661–686. https://doi.org/10.1016/j.compedu.2012.03.004

Creutzig, F., & Kapmeier, F. (2020). Engage, don't preach: Active learning triggers climate action. *Energy Research & Social Science, 70*, 101779. https://doi.org/10.1016/j.erss.2020.101779

Dadaczynski, K., Tolks, D., Wrona, K. J., Mc Call, T., & Fischer, F. (2023). The untapped potential of Games for Health in times of crises. A critical reflection. *Frontiers in Public Health, 11*, 1140665. https://doi.org/10.3389/fpubh.2023.1140665

Damaševičius, R., Maskeliūnas, R., & Blažauskas, T. (2023). Serious games and gamification in healthcare: a meta-review. *Information, 14*, 105. https://doi.org/10.3390/info14020105

Derksen, M. E., Van Strijp, S., Kunst, A. E., Daams, J. G., Jaspers, M. W., & Fransen, M. P. (2020). Serious games for smoking prevention and cessation: A systematic review of game elements and game effects. *Journal of the American Medical Informatics Association, 27*, 818–833. https://doi.org/10.1093/jamia/ocaa013

De Meyer, K., Coren, E., McCaffrey, M., & Slean, C. (2020). Transforming the stories we tell about climate change: from 'issue' to 'action'. *Environmental Research Letters, 16*, 015002. https://doi.org/10.1088/1748-9326/abcd5a

De Salas, K., Ashbarry, L., Seabourne, M., Lewis, I., Wells, L., Dermoudy, J., Roehrer, E., Springer, M., Sauer, J. D., & Scott, J. (2022). Improving environmental outcomes with games: an exploration of behavioural and technological design and evaluation approaches. *Simulation & Gaming*, *53*, 470–512. https://doi.org/10.1177/10468781221114160

DeSmet, A., Van Ryckeghem, D., Compernolle, S., Baranowski, T., Thompson, D., Crombez, G., Poels, K., Van Lippevelde, W., Bastiaensens, S., Van Cleemput, K., Vandebosch, H., & De Bourdeaudhuij, I. (2014). A meta-analysis of serious digital games for healthy lifestyle promotion. *Preventive Medicine*, *69*, 95–107. https://doi.org/10.1016/j.ypmed.2014.08.026

Eskreis-Winkler, L., Troncoso Peres, L. T., & Fishbach, A. (2025). The bigger the problem the littler: When the scope of a problem makes it seem less dangerous. *Journal of Personality and Social Psychology*, 128, 790–806. https://doi.org/10.1037/pspa0000409

Fernández Galeote, D., & Hamari, J. (2021). Game-based climate change engagement: analyzing the potential of entertainment and serious games. *Proceedings of the ACM on Human-Computer Interaction*, *5*, 1–21. https://doi.org/10.1145/3474653

Fernández Galeote, D., Rajanen, M., Rajanen, D., Legaki, N. Z., Langley, D. J., & Hamari, J. (2021). Gamification for climate change engagement: review of corpus and future agenda. *Environmental Research Letters*, *16*, 063004. https://doi.org/10.1088/1748-9326/abec05

Fernández Galeote, D., Legaki, N.-Z., & Hamari, J. (2023). Text-and game-based communication for climate change attitude, self-efficacy, and behavior: A controlled experiment. *Computers in Human Behavior*, 107930. https://doi.org/10.1016/j.chb.2023.107930

Fizek, S., Fiadotau, M., Wirman, H., & Garda, M. (2023). Teaching environmentally conscious game design: Lessons and challenges. *ACM Games: Research and Practice*, *1*, 1–9. https://doi.org/10.1145/3583058

Fjællingsdal, K. S., & Klöckner, C. A. (2019). Gaming green: the educational potential of Eco – a digital simulated ecosystem. *Frontiers in Psychology*, *10*, 2846. https://doi.org/10.3389/fpsyg.2019.02846

Fletcher, R. (2017). Gaming conservation: Nature 2.0 confronts nature-deficit disorder. *Geoforum*, *79*, 153–162. https://doi.org/10.1016/j.geoforum.2016.02.009

Fox, J., McKnight, J., Sun, Y., Maung, D., & Crawfis, R. (2020). Using a serious game to communicate risk and minimize psychological distance regarding environmental pollution. *Telematics and Informatics*, 46, 101320. https://doi.org/10.1016/j.tele.2019.101320

Gao, Z., Pope, Z. C., Lee, J. E., & Quan, M. (2019). Effects of active video games on children's psychosocial beliefs and school day energy expenditure. *Journal of Clinical Medicine*, 8, 1268. https://doi.org/10.3390/jcm8091268

Gampell, A. V., & Gaillard, J. C. (2016). Stop disasters 2.0: Video games as tools for disaster risk reduction. *International Journal of Mass Emergencies & Disasters*, 34, 283–316.

Georgiou, Y., Hadjichambis, A. C., Paraskeva-Hadjichambi, D., & Adamou, A. (2023). "From Gamers into Environmental Citizens": A systematic literature review of empirical research on behavior change games for environmental citizenship. *Multimodal Technologies and Interaction*, *7*, 80. https://doi.org/10.3390/mti7080080

Gerber, A., Ulrich, M., Wäger, F. X., Roca-Puigròs, M., Gonçalves, J. S., & Wäger, P. (2021). Games on climate change: Identifying development potentials through advanced classification and game characteristics mapping. *Sustainability*, *13*, 1997. https://doi.org/10.3390/su13041997

Gifford, R. (2011). The dragons of inaction: psychological barriers that limit climate change mitigation and adaptation. *American Psychologist*, *66*, 290–302. https://psycnet.apa.org/doi/10.1037/a0023566

Greipl, S., Moeller, K., & Ninaus, M. (2020). Potential and limits of game-based learning. *International Journal of Technology Enhanced Learning*, *12*, 363–389. https://doi.org/10.1504/IJTEL.2020.110047

Hall, G., Laddu, D. R., Phillips, S. A., Lavie, C. J., and Arena, R. (2020). A tale of two pandemics: How will COVID-19 and global trends in physical inactivity and sedentary behavior affect one another? *Progress in Cardiovascular Diseases*, 64, 108–110. https://doi.org/10.1016/j.pcad.2020.04.005

Hammady, R., & Arnab, S. (2022). Serious gaming for behaviour change: A systematic review. *Information*, *13*, 142. https://doi.org/10.3390/info13030142

IPCC (2023). Sections. In: Core Writing Team, H. Lee and J. Romero (eds.). *Climate change 2023: Synthesis report. Contribution of working groups I, II and III to the sixth assessment report of the Intergovernmental Panel on Climate Change* (pp. 35–115). IPCC, Geneva, Switzerland. https://10.59327/IPCC/AR6-9789291691647

Kasdorf, R. (2023). Representation of mental illness in video games beyond stigmatization. *Frontiers in Human Dynamics*. 5, 1155821. https://doi.org/10.3389/fhumd.2023.1155821

Kelly, M. (2021). Designing game-based writing projects to foster critical ethical reasoning in the English Classroom: a case study Using Plague Inc: Evolved. *Simulation & Gaming*, 52, 153–168.

Kermavnar, T., Visch, V. T., & Desmet, P. M. (2023). Games in times of a pandemic: structured overview of COVID-19 serious games. *JMIR Serious Games*, *11*, e41766. https://doi.org/10.2196/41766

Khraishah, H., Alahmad, B., Ostergard Jr, R. L., AlAshqar, A., Albaghdadi, M., Vellanki, N., Chowdhury, M. M., Al-Kindi, S. G., Zanobetti, A., Gasparrini, A., & Rajagopalan, S. (2022). Climate change and cardiovascular disease: implications for global health. *Nature Reviews Cardiology*, 19, 798–812. https://doi.org/10.1038/s41569-022-00720-x

Koroleva, K., & Novak, J. (2020). How to engage with sustainability issues we rarely experience? A gamification model for collective awareness platforms in water-related sustainability. *Sustainability*, *12*, 712. https://doi.org/10.3390/su12020712

Krath, J., Schürmann, L., & Von Korflesch, H. F. (2021). Revealing the theoretical basis of gamification: A systematic review and analysis of theory in research on gamification, serious games and game-based learning. *Computers in Human Behavior*, *125*, 106963. https://doi.org/10.1016/j.chb.2021.106963

Kuipers, D. A., Terlouw, G., Wartena, B. O., van't Veer, J. T., Prins, J. T., & Pierie, J. P. E. (2017). The role of transfer in designing games and simulations for health: systematic review. *JMIR Serious Games*, *5*, e7880. https://doi.org/10.2196/games.7880

Lange, F. (2023). Behavioral paradigms for studying pro-environmental behavior: A systematic review. *Behavior Research Methods*, *55*, 600–622. https://doi.org/10.3758/s13428-022-01825-4

Lange, F., & Dewitte, S. (2019). Measuring pro-environmental behavior: Review and recommendations. *Journal of Environmental Psychology*, 63, 92–100. https://doi.org/10.1016/j.jenvp.2019.04.009

Lee, Y. H. (2015). Does digital game interactivity always promote self-efficacy? *Cyberpsychology, Behavior, and Social Networking*, *18*, 669–673. https://doi.org/10.1089/cyber.2015.0165

Maibach, E. W., Nisbet, M., Baldwin, P., Akerlof, K., & Diao, G. (2010). Reframing climate change as a public health issue: an exploratory study of public reactions. *BMC Public Health*, *10*, 1–11. https://doi.org/10.1186/1471-2458-10-299

Malone, R. E., & Proctor, R. N. (2022). Prohibition no, abolition yes! Rethinking how we talk about ending the cigarette epidemic. *Tobacco Control*, *31*, 376–381. https://doi.org/10.1136/tobaccocontrol-2021-056577

Marselle, M. R., Hartig, T., Cox, D. T., De Bell, S., Knapp, S., Lindley, S., Triguero-Mas, M., Böhning-Gaese, K., Braubach, M., Cook, P. A., de Vries, S., Heintz-Buschart, A., Hofmann, M., Irvine, K. N., Kabisch, N., Kolek, F., Kraemer, R, Markevych, I., Martens, D. ... Bonn, A. (2021). Pathways linking biodiversity to human health: A conceptual framework. *Environment International*, *150*, 106420. https://doi.org/10.1016/j.envint.2021.106420

Mayer, I., Bekebrede, G., Harteveld, C., Warmelink, H., Zhou, Q., Van Ruijven, T., Lo, J., Kortmann, R., & Wenzler, I. (2014). The research and evaluation of serious games: Toward a comprehensive methodology. *British Journal of Educational Technology*, *45*, 502–527. https://doi.org/10.1111/bjet.12067

Meriläinen, M., Aurava, R., Kultima, A., & Stenros, J. (2020). Game jams for learning and teaching: a review. *International Journal of Game-Based Learning (IJGBL)*, *10*, 54–71. https://doi.org/10.4018/IJGBL.2020040104

Micallef, D., Parker, L., Brennan, L., Schivinski, B., & Jackson, M. (2022). Improving the health of emerging adult gamers – A scoping review of influences. *Nutrients, 14*, 2226. https://doi.org/10.3390/nu14112226

Moller, A. C., Sousa, C. V., Lee, K. J., Alon, D., & Lu, A. S. (2023). Active Video Game Interventions Targeting Physical Activity Behaviors: Systematic Review and Meta-analysis. *Journal of Medical Internet Research, 25*, e45243. https://doi.org/10.2196/45243

Ndulue, C., & Orji, R. (2022). Games for change – A comparative systematic review of persuasive strategies in games for behaviour change. *IEEE Transactions on Games, 15*, 121–133. https://doi.org/10.1109/TG.2022.3159090

Newzoo (2023). *Global Games Market Report 2023*. https://newzoo.com/resources/trend-reports/newzoo-global-games-market-report-2023-free-version

Newzoo (2025). *Global Games Market Report 2025*. https://newzoo.com/resources/trend-reports/newzoo-global-games-market-report-2025

Ntoumanis, N., Ng, J. Y., Prestwich, A., Quested, E., Hancox, J. E., Thøgersen-Ntoumani, C., Deci, E. L., Ryan, R. M., Lonsdale, C., & Williams, G. C. (2021). A meta-analysis of self-determination theory-informed intervention studies in the health domain: Effects on motivation, health behavior, physical, and psychological health. *Health Psychology Review, 15*, 214–244. https://doi.org/10.1080/17437199.2020.1718529

Onencan, A. M., & Van de Walle, B. (2018). From paris agreement to action: Enhancing climate change familiarity and situation awareness. *Sustainability, 10*, 1929. https://doi.org/10.3390/su10061929

Op de Beke, L., Raessens, J., Werning, S., & Farca, G. (Eds.) (2024). *Ecogames: Playful Perspectives on the Climate Crisis*. Amsterdam University Press.

Ouariachi, T., Olvera-Lobo, M. D., Gutiérrez-Pérez, J., & Maibach, E. (2019). A framework for climate change engagement through video games. *Environmental Education Research, 25*, 701–716. https://doi.org/10.1080/13504622.2018.1545156

Ouariachi, T., Li, C. Y., & Elving, W. J. (2020). Gamification approaches for education and engagement on pro-environmental behaviors: Searching for best practices. *Sustainability, 12*, 4565. https://doi.org/10.3390/su12114565

Palinkas, L. A., & Wong, M. (2020). Global climate change and mental health. *Current Opinion in Psychology, 32*, 12–16. https://doi.org/10.1016/j.copsyc.2019.06.023

Partelow, S., Winkler, K. J., & Thaler, G. M. (2020). Environmental non-governmental organizations and global environmental discourse. *Plos One, 15*, e0232945. https://doi.org/10.1371/journal.pone.0232945

Pathak, M., Slade, R., Shukla, P.R., Skea, J., Pichs-Madruga, R. & Ürge-Vorsatz, D. (2022). Technical Summary. In: P.R. Shukla, J. Skea, R. Slade, A. Al Khourdajie, R. van Diemen, D. McCollum, M. Pathak, S. Some, P. Vyas, R. Fradera, M. Belkacemi, A. Hasija, G. Lisboa, S. Luz, J. Malley, (eds.). *Climate Change 2022: Mitigation of Climate Change. Contribution of Working Group III to the Sixth Assessment Report of the Intergovernmental Panel on Climate Change*. Cambridge University Press, Cambridge, UK and New York, NY, USA. https://10.1017/9781009157926.002

Peng, W. (2008). The mediational role of identification in the relationship between experience mode and self-efficacy: Enactive role-playing versus passive observation. *CyberPsychology & Behavior, 11*, 649–652. https://doi.org/10.1089/cpb.2007.0229

Plass, J. L., Mayer, R. E., & Homer, B. D. (2020). *Handbook of game-based learning*. MIT Press.

Proulx, J. N., Romero, M., & Arnab, S. (2017). Learning mechanics and game mechanics under the perspective of self-determination theory to foster motivation in digital game based learning. *Simulation & Gaming, 48*, 81–97. https://doi.org/10.1177/1046878116674399

Razali, N. E. M., Ramli, R. Z., Mohamed, H., Zin, N. A. M., Rosdi, F., & Diah, N. M. (2022). Identifying and validating game design elements in serious game guideline for climate change. *Heliyon, 8*. https://doi.org/10.1016/j.heliyon.2022.e08773

Rüth, M. (2017). Spielerisches Lernen besser bewerten: Effektivität und Effizienz von Computerspielen [Better evaluation of game-based learning: on effectiveness and efficiency of video gaming]. In: W. Zielinski, S. Aßmann, K. Kaspar, & P. Moormann (Hrsg.), *Spielend lernen! Computerspiele(n) in Schule und Unterricht – Schriftenreihe zur digitalen Gesellschaft NRW (Band 5) [Game-based learning! Video games in school and school teaching. Publication series of the digital society NRW (vol. 5)]* (39–53). München: kopaed.

Rüth, M., & Kaspar, K. (2017). The E-Learning Setting Circle: First steps toward theory development in e-learning research. *The Electronic Journal of e-Learning, 15*, 94–103. https://academic-publishing.org/index.php/ejel/article/view/1822

Rüth, M. (2022). *Learning and teaching with video games. Toward theoretical progress and educational practice* [dissertation]. Köln: Kölner UniversitätsPublikationsServer. http://kups.ub.uni-koeln.de/id/eprint/52965

Rüth, M. (2025). Games, was können wir aus euren Erzählungen lernen? Über die Rolle von Erzählungen beim Lernen mit digitalen Spielen [Games, what can we learn from your narratives? On the role of narratives in learning with digital games] in: M. Kramer, L. Rittiens, K. Schütze, & C. Vollmert (eds.). *Bildung des Narrativen. Transdisziplinäre Perspektiven auf intermediales Erzählen [in] der Postdigitalität* [Formation of the narrative. Transdisciplinary perspectives on Intermedial storytelling [in] Postdigitality] (pp. 205–222). München: Kopaed.

Rüth, M., Bachmayer R., & Kaspar, K. (2025). Learning about depression by watching gaming videos: a case study on the potential of digital games for psychoeducation and destigmatization. *Frontiers in Psychology*, 16, 1585571. https://doi.org/10.3389/fpsyg.2025.1585571

Rüth, M., & Kaspar, K. (2020). Exergames in formal school teaching: A pre-post longitudinal field study on the effects of a dance game on motor learning, physical enjoyment, and learning motivation. *Entertainment Computing, 35*, 100372. https://doi.org/10.1016/j.entcom.2020.100372

Rüth, M., & Kaspar, K. (2021a). Educational and Social Exergaming: A perspective on physical, social, and educational benefits and pitfalls of exergaming at home during the COVID-19 pandemic and afterwards. *Frontiers in Psychology, 12*, 644036. https://doi.org/10.3389/fpsyg.2021.644036

Rüth, M., & Kaspar, K. (2021b). Commercial video games in school teaching: Two mixed methods case studies on students' reflection processes. *Frontiers in Psychology, 11*, 594013. https://doi.org/10.3389/fpsyg.2020.594013

Rüth, M., Schmelzer, M., Burtniak, K., & Kaspar, K (2023). Commercial exergames for rehabilitation of physical health and quality of life: a systematic review of randomized controlled trials with adults in unsupervised home environments. *Frontiers in Psychology, 14*, 1155569. https://doi.org/10.3389/fpsyg.2023.1155569

Sailer, M., Hense, J. U., Mayr, S. K., & Mandl, H. (2017). How gamification motivates: An experimental study of the effects of specific game design elements on psychological need satisfaction. *Computers in Human Behavior, 69*, 371–380. https://doi.org/10.1016/j.chb.2016.12.033

Schunk, D. H., & DiBenedetto, M. K. (2020). Motivation and social cognitive theory. *Contemporary Educational Psychology, 60*, 101832. https://doi.org/10.1016/j.cedpsych.2019.101832

Spangenberger, P., Freytag, S. C., & Geiger, S. M. (2024). Embodying nature in immersive virtual reality: Are multisensory stimuli vital to affect nature connectedness and pro-environmental behaviour? *Computers & Education, 212*, 104964. https://doi.org/10.1016/j.compedu.2023.104964

Speelman, E. N., Escano, E., Marcos, D., & Becu, N. (2023). Serious games and citizen science; from parallel pathways to greater synergies. *Current Opinion in Environmental Sustainability, 64*, 101320. https://doi.org/10.1016/j.cosust.2023.101320

Staiano, A. E., Beyl, R. A., Hsia, D. S., Katzmarzyk, P. T., & Newton Jr, R. L. (2017). Twelve weeks of dance exergaming in overweight and obese adolescent girls: Transfer effects on physical activity, screen time, and self-efficacy. *Journal of Sport and Health Science, 6*, 4–10. https://doi.org/10.1016/j.jshs.2016.11.005

Tian, H., & Liu, X. (2022). Pro-environmental behavior research: Theoretical progress and future directions. *International Journal of Environmental Research and Public Health, 19*, 6721. https://doi.org/10.3390/ijerph19116721

Ubisoft (2021). DevBlog: Eden Burning – The Green Game Jam Scenario. https://anno-union.com/devblog-eden-burning-green-game-jam/

van Valkengoed, A. M., & Steg, L. (2019). Meta-analyses of factors motivating climate change adaptation behaviour. *Nature Climate Change*, *9*, 158–163. https://doi.org/10.1038/s41558-018-0371-y

Vansteenkiste, M., Ryan, R. M., & Soenens, B. (2020). Basic psychological need theory: Advancements, critical themes, and future directions. *Motivation and Emotion*, *44*, 1–31. https://doi.org/10.1007/s11031-019-09818-1

Vervoort, J. M., Milkoreit, M., van Beek, L., Mangnus, A. C., Farrell, D., McGreevy, S. R., Ota, K., Rupprecht, C. D. D., Reed, J. B., & Huber, M. (2022). Not just playing: The politics of designing games for impact on anticipatory climate governance. *Geoforum*, *137*, 213–221. https://doi.org/10.1016/j.geoforum.2022.03.009

Wemyss, D., Cellina, F., Lobsiger-Kägi, E., De Luca, V., & Castri, R. (2019). Does it last? Long-term impacts of an app-based behavior change intervention on household electricity savings in Switzerland. *Energy Research & Social Science*, *47*, 16–27. https://doi.org/10.1016/j.erss.2018.08.018

White, K., Habib, R., & Hardisty, D. J. (2019). How to SHIFT consumer behaviors to be more sustainable: A literature review and guiding framework. *Journal of Marketing*, *83*, 22–49. https://doi.org/10.1177/0022242919825649

Willmott, T., & Rundle-Thiele, S. (2021). Are we speaking the same language? Call for action to improve theory application and reporting in behaviour change research. *BMC Public Health*, *21*, 1–8. https://doi.org/10.1186/s12889-021-10541-1

World Economic Forum (WEF) (2023). *The Global Risks Report 2023*. https://www3.weforum.org/docs/WEF_Global_Risks_Report_2023.pdf

World Economic Forum (WEF) (2025). *The Global Risks Report 2025*. https://reports.weforum.org/docs/WEF_Global_Risks_Report_2025.pdf

World Health Organization (WHO) (2013). *Protecting health from climate change: vulnerability and adaptation assessment*. https://apps.who.int/iris/handle/10665/104200

World Health Organization (WHO) (2021). *Basic documents (49th ed.)*. https://apps.who.int/gb/bd/

World Health Organization (WHO) (2023). *World health statistics 2023: monitoring health for the SDGs, sustainable development goals*. https://www.who.int/publications/i/item/9789240074323

Wu, J. S., & Lee, J. J. (2015). Climate change games as tools for education and engagement. *Nature Climate Change*, *5*, 413–418. https://doi.org/10.1038/nclimate2566

Wyss, A. M., Knoch, D., & Berger, S. (2022). When and how pro-environmental attitudes turn into behavior: The role of costs, benefits, and self-control. *Journal of Environmental Psychology*, *79*, 101748. https://doi.org/10.1016/j.jenvp.2021.101748

Yien, J. M., Hung, C. M., Hwang, G. J., & Lin, Y. C. (2011). A game-based learning approach to improving students' learning achievements in a Nutrition course. *Turkish Online Journal of Educational Technology-TOJET*, *10*, 1–10.

Yuriev, A., Dahmen, M., Paillé, P., Boiral, O., & Guillaumie, L. (2020). Pro-environmental behaviors through the lens of the theory of planned behavior: A scoping review. *Resources, Conservation and Recycling*, *155*, 104660. https://doi.org/10.1016/j.resconrec.2019.104660

Zayeni, D., Raynaud, J. P., & Revet, A. (2020). Therapeutic and preventive use of video games in child and adolescent psychiatry: a systematic review. *Frontiers in Psychiatry*, *11*, 36. https://doi.org/10.3389/fpsyt.2020.00036

# A Psycho-Sociology of Virtualization

## Understanding Hikikomori with Video Games

*Richy Srirachanikorn*

*Hikikomori*, a social issue first popularized in Japan 27 years ago by Saitō Tamaki (1998), rose in prevalence as extreme social withdrawal emerged as a silent epidemic (Silić et al., 2019) during the COVID-19 pandemic (Roza, Furuhashi, & McLeod, 2020). Psychological research falls short in understanding Hikikomori due to its lack of studies, leading to the difficulty of establishing a primary method of intervention (Roza et al., 2021). Given that nostalgic media featured in how people coped with time loss and loneliness during lockdown (Wulf, Breuer, & Schmitt, 2022), and with Svetlana Boym's (2001) wisdom that one is nostalgic for the "past not for the way it was, but for the past the way it could have been" (p. 351), this chapter focuses on the nostalgic potential of one game demo titled HIKIKOMORI LIFE (Micro Team Games, 2022). The chapter wishes to highlight how HIKIKOMORI LIFE, and video games like it, can act as a bridge of "real communication" (Saitō, 1998, p. 84) between its players – parents, psychologists, and the public – whose familiar experiences of being confined at home during COVID-19 and their feelings of nostalgia may aggregate into collective action around this understudied and personal phenomenon. Sociologically, the game operates as an object of nostalgia, allowing players to reflect on how they may try to play the Hikikomori character out of a socially withdrawn past "not for the way it was but for the past the way it could have been" (Boym, 2001, p. 351). Whilst the video game, an object for nostalgia that allows non-Hikikomori players to play the Hikikomori character towards a past that could have been lived if not for social withdrawal, the subject of the Hikikomori operates as a nostalgic object, fettered by psychological literature and media portrayals that makes up the past that was prescribed to them. To untangle this, the analysis borrows from Sloan (2016), whose "games-on-games" (p. 42) methodology is reapplied to our own personal and collective memories of Hikikomori. Ultimately, I will propose a psycho-sociology of virtualization: one part being *virtual* in the technology it deals with and employs, whilst the other is an imaginative effort by the potential players of HIKIKOMORI LIFE whose common nostalgic feelings as evoked by the game may help forward the virtualization (Lévy, 1995) of a past for the way it could have been.

## "Home" sickness

Nostalgia translates from the Greek *nostos*, as going home, and *algos*, as pain. Arguably, video games possess both of these qualities by allowing adult players to revisit their childhood memories where these games were played physically at home. In terms of pain, the realization that the life associated with this childhood home no longer exists in the present day is what Boym (2001) calls reflective nostalgia, which is "a form of deep mourning that performs a labour of grief both through pondering pain and through play that points the future" (p. 55). Although Boym did not believe that computers could capture the virtualities of the human imagination (p. 50), they are nonetheless apt tools that can converge the imaginations of multiple individuals who are in pain, longing for "home". This form of nostalgic play therefore utilizes video games as digital time machines (Wulf et al., 2018), which may help non-and-Hikikomori alike to realize the past that was lost (Roza et al., 2020) into the past "for the way it could have been" (Boym, 2001, p. 351).

However, "home" may also exist as a metaphorical space, where participants were able to feel nostalgic without the prompt of physical game consoles, but by just remembering gaming experiences (Wulf et al., 2018). With what did they use to draw this nostalgia from? During lockdown, these were the lucrative nostalgic media services such as Disney+, revived online video games such as WORLD OF WARCRAFT CLASSIC (Robinson & Bowman, 2022), and a mix of retro content inside futuristic machines like the Nintendo Switch, which sold over 28.3 million units by the end of 2020 alone (Owens, 2022). Metaphorically, it is a "return home... [even] if it's not your home; by the time you reach it, you will have already forgotten the difference" (Boym, 2001, p. 44). This form of restorative nostalgia (Boym, 2001) operates as "collective memory [which] is seen as a playground, not as a graveyard of multiple individual recollections" (p. 54). Nostalgia can therefore be understood sociologically, where what is no longer present in the individual's life, due to the natural passing of time or from opportunity cost, becomes a rare object or valued highly based on the definitions of a collective home (Niemeyer and Keightley 2020). This "home" built by collective memory perpetuates a nostalgia that is not a pursuit of personal loss, but a loss that is personalized by a collective. Yet, for Hikikomori, how can they rely on a restorative time that 'could be' if 'what was' reflective is still what they are living and remain in? Who can they turn to miss if the same individuals who should be their support system also perpetuate the "structural ignorance" (Saito, 1998, p. 17) of taboo surrounding the social withdrawal?

## Playing with the past

Recently, Roza and colleagues (2021) reminded pandemic researchers about Hikikomori, a term popularized by Japanese psychologist Saitō Tamaki (1998) describing adolescents to middle-aged adults who have severely withdrawn from social life for over six months. With the COVID-19 pandemic, previously noted international cases of Hikikomori have magnified from a silent epidemic (Silić et al., 2019) into one whereby "strict confinement measures may have... increase[d] the time spent gaming or on the Internet" (Roza et al., 2021, p. 115). Accordingly, these actions were positively associated with a higher risk of developing Hikikomori (Gavin & Brosnan, 2022) in addition to being male and not leaving home for long periods of time, both established as conventional factors in psychological literature (Dziesinski, 2008; Teo, 2010).

Popular media depictions of Hikikomori as a paranoic protagonist who believes that he is being played by a widespread conspiracy in *Welcome to the N.H.K.* (2002), to the violent and unstable antagonist who chooses to stay in the desolate 'game world' of *Alice in Borderland (2020–2022)* perpetuate the notion that these are individuals who choose to socially withdraw because of games. Relatedly, a quick search of "Hikikomori" on the Steam store website reveals the trailers to 4 video games: two titles task the player to play as or to protect a Hikikomori against neighbors, martial art bandits, and robots (Blaze Epic, 2016; Nito Souji, 2025). Conversely, *Dream of the Hikikomori* (Whittaker, 2022) pits the unattractive player with disadvantages against a slew of characters in a dating simulator. Ultimately, the life of the Hikikomori is treated as a being confined or equated to a game; it is not serious enough to escape the entire fantasy of the situation. Such determinism is similar to Tisseron's (2004) argument that engaging into the world of video games is inevitable as Hikikomori realizes that their expectations of the real world do not match their experience and abilities to realize them. A recent account of Hikikomori has supported this claim when the individual played so intensely to "the point that the real world lost meaning and significance" (Silić et al., 2019, p. 321). Consequently, media depictions echo scholarly arguments that propose it is media which is the cause of withdrawal (Adamski, 2018; Stip et al., 2016). As such, these texts portray Hikikomori as "youth both 'at risk', and a 'risk to'" (Berman & Rizzo, 2019) others, based on a 'past that was' and continues to be prescribed by the collective memory of media and scholarly depiction. This is what Boym (2001) calls a restorative nostalgic understanding of time because its fixation on a past informed by technological determinism "does not help us to deal with the future" (p. 351).

Hence, the fourth game of Hikikomori Life by Micro Team Games (2022) is chosen for analysis. It depicts a Hikikomori confined at home, timeless; all that exists is the player, the character, and the present. Promisingly, the game is still in demo, meaning that the project is not completely built as a restorative recollection of

Hikikomori. On the Steam website's description, the game wants its players to experience and be educated about "the hard life of a game addict. [To] Feel the loneliness if you can. [And] How infuriating it is when everything distracts you. And so [the player will] want to play!" (Micro Team Games, 2022). This collaborative spirit echoes the one shared by Kato, Sartorius, and Shinfuku (2020), whose call to action for the involvement of third parties led to the implementation of an education program for family members surrounding the stigma and taboo of Hikikomori. As such, for the player of HIKIKOMORI LIFE, the tensions between playing to better understand the past for the way it was for the Hikikomori as recalled by media and scholarly memory, whilst trying to play towards a past that could have been to relieve the Hikikomori out of withdrawal, is where the analysis is concerned.

## Life's a game

Split into three sections, I first discuss the ostensibly simple motivations which players of HIKIKOMORI LIFE must complete as tasks to sustain the played-Hikikomori character (or the "hikan") in the present. However, just as Kato and colleagues (2017) highlight how a video game motivated a socially withdrawn individual out of their past for the way it was, I expose how the game tries to force its own notions for a past the way it could have been better onto the hikan. This will be revealed with the game's complicated motivations behind its ostensibly simple tasks. Secondly, Sloan's (2016) games-on-games method is adopted to showcase a "shattering of nostalgic selectiveness" (p. 42). Whilst HIKIKOMORI LIFE may resemble mechanical and aesthetical nostalgia of previous video games, its subject matter may not have been familiar with the memory of non-Japanese audiences until recent nostalgic media and scholarly attention. Bridging this memory is with the nostalgic encounter of players' previous game experiences and their chronophobia during COVID-19, or the anxiety of not knowing how to meaningfully spend time that is depleting (Boym, 2001). This, along with exposing the game's ulterior motivations, recognizes the nostalgic objects of old game titles and mechanics that HIKIKOMORI LIFE employs to familiarize its non-Japanese players to a topic that has only started to emerge into global attention but remains understudied. How the nostalgic experiences of COVID-19 are evoked by the game, the tensions emerging with the nostalgia of previous video games, and how this all impacts the collective memory of *Hikikomori* is discussed.

## Simple motivations, complicated meanings

When players begin a new game on HIKIKOMORI LIFE, they are situated in a dark, old, apartment complex divided into a studio, a kitchen, a laundry room, and a bathroom. Given the message "Welcome to the hikan simulator! Your task is to satisfy game addiction and not to perish from human needs", players are instructed to keep the Hikikomori character alive by tending to 8 total needs by walking up to an object in the apartment and choosing the appropriate actions.

*Figure 1: Screenshot of* HIKIKOMORI LIFE

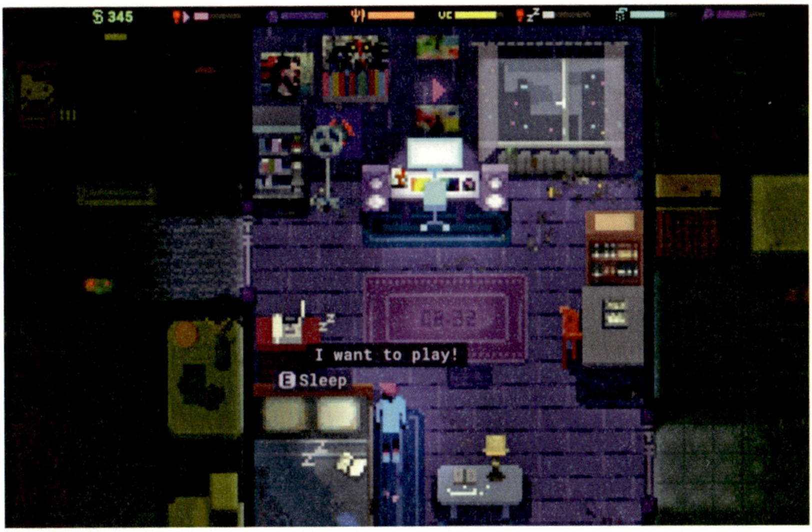


Screenshot by Author

In the game, to fulfill "Money" and "Game Addict" is to use the computer to work or play, the former rewarding money to purchase the maid cleaning service (with the choice to replace them with a robot vacuum) and pest control which fulfills "Purity". Crucially, the only other choice to spend income from hard work on the computer is to upgrade their desktop and to buy more video games, increasing the pink 'needs' meter of "Game Addict". If this need is low or empty, interactions with objects responsible for fulfilling other needs cannot be performed, just as "IF SOMETHING DETTRACTS, IT IS IMPOSSIBLE TO PLAY!!!" (Micro Team Games, 2022). Even with extreme exhaustion, one must satisfy "Game Addict" before their "Need to Sleep" because the character will protest that "I have a gaming bug!", or "I want to play!" (Fig. 1). Once the meter for "Game Addict" is over, so is the life of the hikan character. As such, players must obsess with "satisfy[ing] physiological needs, eliminate distractions [and figure out] how [they] can play, play, play without it." (Micro Team Games, 2022). Achieving this is to play not only as, but *like* a game addict, aligning with one of the game's advertised motivations. What is 'real' about life – physiological needs, social bonds, or 'distractions' – is to be minimized, whilst 'life' itself is accentuated as the primary goal, reflecting the account of Rooksby, Furuhashi, & McLeod (2020) who noted Hikikomori's "aspir[ation] to social death [but] avoiding physical death" (p. 399).

Ironically, in the attempt to keep playing HIKIKOMORI LIFE, the life of the Hikikomori must be played with. When encountering any "random events... [the player must] manage to eliminate [them and] everything" (Micro Team Games, 2022), including the possibility for the Hikikomori character to live their life. The hikan is the extinguisher of goods and items embodying life's problems, not the other way round. As such, the player is tasked to virtualize (Lévy, 1995) by drawing from their second-hand nostalgia. Rather than embracing a 'psychology of the hikan', the game pushes for a restorative 'Hikikomori psychology' by making the life of the hikan the central object which players use to play into the social withdrawal. Consequently, players of HIKIKOMORI LIFE are motivated to virtualize (Lévy, 1995) by overlooking "any relationship with a real object" (Tisseron, 2004, p. 9) such as the household items of the digital apartment that may indicate the nostalgic history or biography of the hikan's past not only for the way it was, but "for the past the way it could have been" (Boym, 2001, p. 351). In essence, the Hikikomori label is prioritized over the human behind it. If fulfilling this motivation fails and the hikan becomes 'distracted', then the player fails at the game because its goal is to "experience the hard life of a hikan suffering from gam[ing] addiction" (Micro Team Games, 2022).

Therefore, the past which could have been is not present in gameplay because players are not given the information or motivation to regard the personal psychology of the hikan, and to later form expectations and behaviors about how to virtualize (Lévy, 1995) towards a way out. Even if players grind away to upgrade the gaming set up or collect great income, the hikan remains with the same set of flashing problems around the house. By trying to demotivate the hikan out of their "Game Addict[ion]", the player's own motivation means that they are not playing the game as intended since the hikan dies. Conversely, players who are motivated to keep the hikan alive by grinding away at upgrades and income do so only to further their addiction, rendering the hikan demotivated from dealing with their social withdrawal by remaining a "Game Addict". Seemingly, there is no way out.

The fundamental issue for the hikan in HIKIKOMORI LIFE is therefore not the game addiction that is hard to break, or the playing of computer games, but the ultimate game that never ends: daily life. Reflexively, the player has to ask herself: what am *I* most motivated to play towards? Is it for a player-centric desire to "experience the hard life of a hikan suffering from gam[ing] addiction" (Micro Team Games, 2022) and to progress in it by forcing the hikan to constantly extinguish the problems of everyday life in their apartment? Or is it for a hikan-centric desire to stop playing the game of life but to dwell in game addiction whilst the player is limited to play the game as it intended? Either way, both avenues are recycled through replays as encouraged by the game to "start...again and try to kill the character in different ways" (Micro Team Games, 2022). Ultimately, for the situation of real-world Hikikomori, the game of life and on the computer never ends because both contain what sociologist Erving Goffman (1969) calls "externally grounded matter[s]" (p. 27) which if left unaddressed, can "have a continuing significance outside the current encounter" (p. 27) or 'game' that is played at the moment. Contemporarily, there are complex but intertwining relationships between video gaming as a risk of developing Hikikomori (Gavin & Brosnan, 2022) or with "hikikomori sufferers [who through playing] may forget their own lonely feelings" (Kato, Shinfuku, & Tateno, 2020, p. 268). Thus, even with researchers, the ostensibly simple motivation to play into or away one's problems is complicated by prioritizing whether the outcome is a treatment or solution. Here, the miniature version of this developing effort in HIKIKOMORI LIFE asks that very complex question to its players.

## Playing with what was always at play

HIKIKOMORI LIFE employs a few nostalgic properties. Observably, its pixelated look borrows from retro-styled games that "older games people [have experienced and] can essentially return to the exact same virtual space that they explored in earlier times" (Wulf et al., 2018, p. 60). In terms of its mechanics, the needs bars and life simulation genre strike up memories of *The Sims* franchise (Electronic Arts, 2000), whose bars (also numbering eight) are virtually the same except for "Room" or "Environment"; the desire for a spacious, lively, and well-decorated habitable area (The Sims wiki, n.d.), and the "Social" meter. As such, players of *Hikikomori Life* may use their reflective nostalgic experiences from *The Sims* to inform gameplay choices or style. To put "games-on-games", according to Sloan (2016, p. 35), is to use our memories of and from the past, as carried by video games, to inform the present. Whilst HIKIKOMORI LIFE does not explicitly declare its retro references, the mere fact that it encourages players to "Experience the hard life of a hikan suffering from gam[ing] addiction" (Micro Team Games, 2022) is enough to qualify it as a form of digital nostalgia (Niemeyer, 2016) which is not to yearn for game consoles or machines, but "the human relations it created" (p. 29). In this case, it is to think about the hikan's possible loneliness in the past and the lack of support from social actors in the present. Hence, prior to being played, *Hikikomori Life* has the "potential... to offer any form of critical engagement with the past" (Sloan, 2016, p. 36) on its own.

On the surface, it may not seem productive to put THE SIMS and HIKIKOMORI LIFE together, since the former does not center on the issue of Hikikomori. They are both life simulators with the former focusing on the rewards of life, such as progression, wealth, and growing one's lineage, and the latter on life's never-ending problems. Comparing the game world of THE SIMS to the real-world space where the playing happens, Wark (2006) points out that both realms are inherently unfulfilling. For Hikikomori, whom Tisseron (2004) believes uses virtual worlds to detach from the real world due to the realization that their expectations can never be met with their abilities, the game world does not offer a permanent solution. In-game cutscenes that will trigger certain events, a game's limited code that allows only so many choices, and upon logging out, the real world that awaits the player are all rules that cannot be bent. These rules are what Alex Galloway (as cited in Wark, 2006) calls allegorithms, which keep the "future… forever promised but [which] never comes to pass" (p. 4). To compare, THE SIMS (TS) and HIKIKOMORI LIFE (HL) possess separate and overlapping allegorithms:

- Upon reaching a certain point of gameplay, a non-rewindable cutscene or trigger appears, forcing a definitive game action: Not tending to the needs of the game character will always result in death (TS/HL), whilst specific needs such as "Game Addiction" (HL) and a child's schooling and social relationships (TS) must be maintained otherwise they will die (HL) or be sent to military school (TS) and suffer a low and red "Social" bar.
- More importantly, allegorithms restrict the player's agency: those who succeeded in becoming wealthy and living in their dream house cannot stamp their legacy by dying there of old age; this is impossible (TS). Players who work tirelessly on the computer to gain income can only spend that money on cleaning services where the only other human is a maid who will never interact with the player, or a robot vacuum (HL). Only money can be spent on computer upgrades and video games in HL to progress into "Game Addiction", and not for therapy or comfier furniture.
- Thus, allegorithms characterize the experience of the game as much as they reflect the gamespace and life itself: no matter how much the game's virtualization can reflect a life or past "that could have been" (Boym, 2001, p. 351), players inside and outside of the game are tangled by time, routine, and mundanity (Wark, 2006).

The real game that never ends – arguably the one that matters most – is how we deal with life itself. Wark's (2006) three certainties of life can be summed up with Boym's (2001) uncertain chronophobia, which is the "disease of the millennium" (p. 351) that is not a fear of time, but a constant anxiety of not knowing how to spend a depletion of it meaningfully. In other words, if the past that was embodies time that is already lost, then the effort to successfully actualize the past for the way it could have been must minimize as much loss as possible. These losses, as I have argued elsewhere (Srirachanikorn forthcoming), are the microtransactions, hoarding, and the chasing of restorative nostalgia that "does not help us to deal with the future"

(Boym, 2001, p. 351). Although the two games diverge in how they approach life – one rewarding life's milestones in spite of its problems (TS) whilst the other rewarding players who perpetuate the problematic lifestyle that is Gaming Addiction (HL) – they converge with the same problem of time. Poignantly, Wark (2006) argued that "The game ties up one loose end with which gamespace struggles—the mortal flaw of an irreversible time." However, even with two decades between the games' releases, HIKIKOMORI LIFE'S "imitation [of life] that is shaped by contemporary perceptions of the past" (Sloan, 2016, p. 38) and THE SIMS retain the same restorative nostalgia that life still has the same eight problems, that we must do whatever it takes to fulfill them, and that time is constantly depleting. Perhaps this "loose end" (Wark, 2006) may work for players whose regrets and events of the pasts are not constantly fettered to their present, or the static world of their room. For Hikikomori, this may become a knot that ties the inability to actualize their expectations (Tisseron, 2004) with further disappointment that virtual machines cannot do this either. Following Wark (2006), "what is true..." (p. 5) as the desires for a past that the Hikikomori wishes could be in the game "...is not real," (p. 5), and "what is real..." (p. 5) as the present-day situation "...is not true." (p. 5) inside the virtuality of the game world. If players accept the current state of affairs, then they are left with a reflective nostalgia to mourn their own depleting needs and desires up until this point in life.

However, HIKIKOMORI LIFE is not a static moment of the past – it is a contemporary digital time machine (Wulf et al., 2018) to get players to "lon[g] for the human relations" (Niemeyer, 2016, p. 29) between the in-game hikan, the non-interacting maid, the loud neighbors and city, and the internet. In other words, players of HIKIKOMORI LIFE are encouraged to be conscious about whether they are playing the past not for the way it was but for the way it could have been. Neither is wrong, because the primary plaything here is not time loss but the gaining of things in spite of time loss. Differing from a pastiche of imitating life passively is what Sloan (2016) identifies as parody, which employs a "shattering of nostalgic selectiveness" (p. 42) in how HIKIKOMORI LIFE does not reward its players the restorative nostalgia of what life could be according to its similar counterpart, THE SIMS. Rather than job promotions, marriage, children, special events, or death by old age, players of HIKIKOMORI LIFE who manage to accumulate great income by consistently working on the computer or by fulfilling all needs are rewarded with the "Demo game time is over. You can start the game again and try to kill the character in different ways." (Micro Team Games, 2022). In other words, there is no future for the hikan not because the game prevents us from progressing into something else, but because in the game's present, the idea of progress by job promotion, death by old age, and social relationships does not exist. It shatters our restorative nostalgic understandings of how one works to better their life, and how a better life works out to be. Whilst the game is indeed still in demo, the potential for such progress to be made through whatever narrative and mechanic presented thus far is convincing that the option for 'a way out' was never there to begin with. What we were playing with was therefore *our* nostalgic restorations about Hikikomori, and *our* experiences of dealing with time loss, and not towards a stage or phase where things get better, or somebody 'wins'. Interestingly, for a thematically progressive game, there was no progress (in how we understand it) in the game to be made. It is up to the player, and the realization that the "real" game that never ends is not the one that is associated with video games that the so-called addicted Hikikomori plays, but the game that everyone has to play: trying to navigate through chronophobia (Boym, 2001) in mundane everyday life.

The real nostalgic potential of HIKIKOMORI LIFE is therefore the reminder that we are not playing towards a better or improved HIKIKOMORI LIFE here; we are playing with the life of a Hikikomori and that is it. We are not in the past that was, but the very present of people who have yet to be understood widely and deeply (Roza et al., 2021). Put simply, "nostalgia should be put into perspective" (Niemeyer, 2016, p. 30) because it will inform how we virtualize interventions and futures for such individuals whose perspectives we truly know very little about.

## Game over? (Conclusion)

In this chapter, I attempted to show how HIKIKOMORI LIFE can operate as a nostalgic object for non-Hikikomori players to look back at their lives with, particularly during the COVID-19 pandemic. More importantly, the game can also become an object of nostalgia that reveals how we are playing with the past that was prescribed, not only to Hikikomori by psychological literature, but also to us, by popular media.

As such, a psycho-sociology of virtualization hopes to pave way for a person-focused, empathetic, and non-clinical nostalgia of the Hikikomori. To do this, it relies on video games to engage with two kinds of virtuality. The first follows Lévy (1995) and Tisseron (2004) in reflecting how we, through the nostalgia that is practiced and purchased, act on our virtual concepts of things, events, and pasts that we wish could have been. This is evident in how we play video games to change or relive our distant pasts from decades ago, by relying on familiar checkmarks of collective memory that may exist in the present, becoming what Makai (2018) calls an effective cultural mediator of history. Second, rather than playing HIKIKOMORI LIFE alone and with the history of a fictional hikan, players who are committed or connected to the subject of Hikikomori should each individually play the game, but do so next to each other. In this way, they are able to engage with their own biographies in the experiences with Hikikomori, their chronophobia (Boym, 2001), feelings of loneliness, and their uses of virtual worlds as a respite. Curiously, Tisseron (2004) also argued that the way Hikikomori plays video games "might represent their attempt to self-healing" (p. 7), pointing to the future that the Hikikomori in the present desires. When applied to HIKIKOMORI LIFE'S non-interactive items inside of the room, players may speculate what the hikan wants for their future. Speculating on the psychology of the Hikikomori can shatter the nostalgic selectiveness of HIKIKOMORI LIFE that perpetuates a restorative Hikikomori psychology attached to a predetermined past that could never be anything else.

This second form of virtuality – or what I will call the *nostalgic potential* – of video games may unite people in their experiences of nostalgia and chronophobia (Boym, 2001) during COVID-19 to sympathize with Hikikomori (Wong, 2020). With this, video games can invert their position from depicting Hikikomori as a nostalgic object of collective memory, to becoming an object for nostalgia to be shared amongst a collective around this extremely personal issue. These implementations not only complement the current efforts to shift attention to the individuals around the Hikikomori, educating family members about the taboo of social withdrawal (Kato, Sartorius, & Shinfuku, 2020), but also speak to the "more proactive approach" (Wong & Li, 2021) that in-game rewards have on the motivation of a Hikikomori to leave their withdrawal (Kato et al., 2017). Games that reward its players may create a rewarding game experience for non-Hikikomori to develop an informed, fun, and united collective. Importantly, this psycho-sociological use of a video game's *nostalgic potential* furthers the intent of Saitō Tamaki (1998), whose insight that the phenomenon stems from a "structural ignorance" (p. 17) which requires an equally structural bond to nurture key factors for treatment: time, informed supporters of the Hikikomori, and "real communication" (p. 84). Video games may very well fit this bill.

Scholars have started to argue for the cultural boundlessness of Hikikomori (Hamasaki et al., 2021), highlighting how a collective effort amongst "psychology, engineering, sociology, and politics" (Kato, Sartorius, & Shinfuku, 2020, p. 1) is imperative for a social problem where its sufferers rarely reach out for help, if at all (Wong & Li, 2021). More so, Kato and colleagues (2017) have found that "Clear and 'realistic' rewards in the world of video games lead to immediate satisfaction" (p. 75) and is thus enticing as a "first step towards more permanent solutions" (p. 75). The game which never ends is therefore the one that requires everyone other than the Hikikomori to *keep* playing their part. In the case of HIKIKOMORI LIFE, by employing a psycho-sociology of virtualization, we can now see that in helping the hikan avoid death, players are ironically prolonging a life not for the way it could be better but "for the way it was" (Boym, 2001, p. 351). This action echoes the sentiment that Rooksby and colleagues (2020) have identified as an "aspir[ation] to social death and avoiding physical death [a]s a core feature of people with hikikomori – they want society to forget them, but they cannot forget society" (p. 399). Given that players and video games will continue to mature together (Wulf et al., 2018) alongside nostalgia and chronophobia as a "human predicament" (Boym, 2001, p. 351) into endless commercial outputs (Niemeyer, 2016), a solution involving the nostalgic potential of video games for a topic such as Hikikomori is an effort that should be personal and personalized – both at the investigation and the response – only because change can be done and experienced in its benefits, collectively.

## References

Adamski, D. (2018). The influence of new technologies on the social withdrawal (hikikomori syndrome) among developed communities, including Poland. *Social communication, 1*, 58–63. https://doi.org/10.2478/sc-2018-0007

Berman, N., & Rizzo, F. (2019). Unlocking Hikikomori: An interdisciplinary approach. *Journal of Youth Studies, 22*(6), 791–806. https://doi.org/10.1080/13676261.2018.1544416

Blaze Epic. (2016). HIKIKOMORI NO CHUUNIBYOU. [PC]. Steam. https://store.steampowered.com/app/501940/Hikikomori_No_Chuunibyou/

Boym, S. (2001). *The future of nostalgia*. Basic Books. Dziesinski, M. (2008). From failed sons to working men: Rehabilitating hikikomori. Presented at the *American Sociological Association Annual Meeting*.

Electronic Arts. (2000). THE SIMS. [Multiple Platforms].

Gavin, J. & Brosnan, M. (2022). The relationship between hikikomori risk and internet use during COVID-19 restrictions. *Cyberpsychology, behavior, and social networking, 25*(3), 189–193. https://doi.org/10.1089/cyber.2021.0171.

Goffman, E. (1961). Fun in games. In Encounters: Two studies in the sociology of interaction. (Pp. 15–72). Indianapolis: Bobbs-Merrill.

Hamasaki, Y., Pionnié-Dax, N., Dorard, G., Tajan, N., & Hikida, T. (2021). Identifying social withdrawal (Hikikomori) factors in adolescents: Understanding the Hikikomori spectrum. *Child Psychiatry Hum Dev 52*, 808817. https://doi.org/10.1007/s10578-020-01064-8

Kato, T. A., Sartorius, N., & Shinfuku, N. (2020). Forced social isolation due to COVID-19 and consequent mental health problems; Lessons from *hikikomori*. *Psychiatry and clinical neurosciences, 74*(9), 506–507. https://doi.org/10.1111/pcn.13112

Kato, T. A., Shinfuku, N., & Tateno, M. (2020). Internet society, internet addiction, and pathological social withdrawal: The chicken and egg dilemma for internet addiction and hikikomori. *Current Opinion in Psychiatry, 33*(3), 264–270. https://doi.org/10.1097/YCO.0000000000000601

Kato, T. A., Teo, A. R., Tateno, M., Watabe, M., Kubo, H., & Kanba, S. (2017). Can Pokémon GO rescue shut-ins (hikikomori) from their isolated world? *Psychiatry and clinical neurosciences, 71*, 70–76. https://doi.org/ 10.1111/pcn.12481

Lévy, P. (1995). Becoming virtual: Reality in the digital age. New York: Plenum Press.

Makai, P. K. (2018). Video games as objects and vehicles of nostalgia. *Humanities, 7*(4), 123. https://doi.org/10.3390/h7040123

Micro Team Games. (2022). HIKIKOMORI LIFE. [PC]. Steam. https://store.steampowered.com/app/1597800/Hikikomori_life/

Niemeyer, K. (2016). Digital nostalgia. *Media Development, 4*, 27–30.

Niemeyer, K., & Keightley, E. (2020). The commodification of time and memory: Online communities and the dynamics of commercially produced nostalgia. *New Media & Society, 22*(9), 1639–1662. https://doi.org/10.1177/1461444820914869

Nito Souji. (2025). PULL STAY. Steam. https://store.steampowered.com/app/1179890/Pull_Stay/

Owens, T. (2022, August 11). Annual sales of Nintendo Switch worldwide 2017–2021. *Statista*. https://www.statista.com/statistics/1085606/annual-unit-sales-nintendo-switchworldwide/#: :text=Annual%20sales%20of%20Nintendo%20Switch%20worldwide%202017%2D2021&text=Sales%20continued%20to%20increase%20in,close%20rival%2C%20Microsoft's%20Xbox%20One

Robinson, J. A., & Bowman, N. D. (2022). Returning to Azeroth: Nostalgia, sense of place, and social presence in World of Warcraft Classic. *Games and culture: A journal of interactive media, 17*(3), 421–444. https://doi.org/10.1177/15554120211034759.

Rooksby, M., Furuhashi, T., & McLeod, H. (2020). Hikikomori: A hidden mental health need following the COVID-19 pandemic. *World psychiatry, 19*(3), 399–400. https://doi.org/10.1002/wps.20804.

Roza, T. H., Spritzer, D. T., Gadelha, A., & Passos, I. C. (2021). *Hikikomori* and the COVID-19 pandemic: Not leaving behind the socially withdrawn. *Brazilian journal of psychiatry, 43*, 114–116. http://dx.doi.org/10.1590/15164446-2020-1145

Saitō, T. (1998). *Hikikomori: adolescence without end*. University of Minnesota Press. Retrieved April 30 2023 from http://site.ebrary.com/id/10681173

Silić, A., Vukojević, J., Čulo, I., & Falak, H. (2019). Hikikomori silent epidemic. *Research in psychotherapy: Psychopathology, process and outcome, 22*(2), 317–322. https://doi.org/10.4081/ripppo.2019.377

Sloan, R. (2016). Nostalgia videogames as playable game criticism. *GAME, 5*, 35–45.

Stip, E., Thibault, A., Beauchamp-Chatel, A., & Kisely, S. (2016). Internet addiction, hikikomori syndrome, and the prodromal phase of psychosis. *Front. Psychiatry, 7*(6). https://doi.org/10.3389/fpsyt.2016.00006

Teo A. R. (2010). A new form of social withdrawal in Japan: a review of hikikomori. *The International journal of social psychiatry, 56*(2), 178–185. https://doi.org/10.1177/0020764008100629

The Sims Wiki. (n.d.). Environment. *The Sims Wiki*. https://sims.fandom.com/wiki/Environment.

Tisseron, S. (2004). On psychological virtuality and its hazards: Hikikomori and virtual object relations. *Funzione Gamma*, N. 38, 1–11.

Wark, M. (2006). Digital allegories (on the Sims). (2006). *Grey Room, 25*, 126–138.

Whittaker, S. (2022). DREAM OF THE HIKIKOMORI. [PC]. Steam. https://store.steampowered.com/app/1788560/Dream_Of_The_Hikikomori/.

Wong, P. (2020). Potential changes to the hikikimori phenomenon in the wake of the Covid-19 pandemic. Asian journal of psychiatry, 54, 102288. https://doi.org/10.1016/j.ajp.2020.102288

Wong, P. & Li, T. (2021). Hikikomori: Risks and consequences of extreme self-imposed social marginalization. In R. J. Coplan, J. C. Bowker, & L. J. Nelson (Eds.), *The handbook of solitude: Psychological perspectives on social isolation, social withdrawal, and being alone* (2nd ed.). (pp. 378–389). Wiley-Blackwell.

Wulf, T., Bowman, N. D., Rieger, D., Velez, J. A., & Breuer, J. (2018). Video games as time machines: Video game nostalgia and the success of retro gaming. *Media and Communication*, 6(2), 60–68. https://doi.org/10.17645/mac.v6i2.1317

Wulf, T., Breuer, J., & Schmitt, J. B. (2022). Escaping the pandemic present: The relationship between nostalgic media use, escapism, and well-being during the COVID-19 pandemic. Psychology of popular media, 11(3):258–265. https://doi.org/10.1037/ppm0000357

# Representation

# Good Grief

## What Video Games Teach Us About Loss

*Kelli Dunlap and Christopher Leech*

Grief is a natural reaction to experiencing significant loss. It is often discussed within the context of death—the loss of a loved one—but can also be experienced following non-fatal losses such as the loss of health, loss of financial security, or loss of important interpersonal relationships. In short, anything we have an attachment to can be lost and anything that can be lost can be grieved. Grief and loss are fundamental to the human experience (Hall, 2014), yet despite this universality people are often ill-equipped to navigate grief in themselves or in others (Ivy, 2022; McLean et al., 2022). Social norms frequently dictate that the expression of grief, especially emotional expression (e.g. crying, sadness, distress), be hidden and kept out of sight (though this does vary by factors such as age, race, gender, etc.; James & Friedman, 2017; McLean et al., 2022).These same social norms frequently promote or reinforce myths about grief and contribute to a harmful disconnect between what society deems normal and appropriate and what grieving people actually experience and need (Kahler et al., 2019; McLean et al., 2022).

Talking about or displaying grief in daily life is taboo (Ivy, 2022) but is quite common in the news (Florea & Rabatel, 2011) and in entertainment media (Coward-Gibbs, 2020; Harrer, 2018; Lund, 2022). While some of these representations perpetuate grief myths and harmful social norms, grief portrayals in media can have a powerful impact on normalizing grief, destigmatizing bereavement, confronting and correcting misinformation, and modeling how to navigate the unimaginable (Davis, 2022).

Death, grief, and loss have been core experiences in entertainment media since humans began telling stories. 2,000 years ago, Aristotle wrote about the "paradox of tragedy" wherein audiences enjoyed witnessing misery and pain through tragic theater as a way to purge difficult or unpleasant emotions (catharsis) via a simulated representation that an audience could empathize with (mimesis; Morreall, 1968). And while grief and its expression continue to be taboo in daily life, interest and engagement with grief in popular media has increased in the last decade (Lund, 2022; Jacobsen et al., 2020).

As the dominant media form of the 21st century (Johnson, 2019), video games are excellently positioned and uniquely capable of significantly impacting public experience and understanding, and shifting larger social norms, around grief and loss. This chapter serves as a primer on grief in games for game developers by: 1) providing relevant information about grief and loss from clinical, cultural, and personal perspectives; 2) briefly reviewing of the history of games as a vehicle for accessible and meaningful experiences around death, loss, and grief; 3) analyzing select games designed to evoke feelings of grief in loss in players; and 4) proposing a best practice matrix for ethically and meaningfully including grief into a game's narrative, mechanical, and aesthetic design.

## What are death, loss, and grief?

Grief, death, and loss are irrevocably connected and frequently used interchangeably. While the terms are closely related, they are distinctly separate phenomena. Death refers to the end of life, an irreversible cessation of biological functions required to sustain an organism (Merriam-Webster, n.d.). While death is quite specific, loss is more ambiguous. Loss is defined as having less of, or no longer having, something (Cambridge Dictionary, 2023b). Within the context of this paper, loss can mean loss of life (i.e. death), but can also describe other significant losses such as loss of health, loss of relationships, loss of employment, etc. In other words, death is a loss but not all losses are deaths. Both death and loss are events, things occurring externally to a person. Grief, however, is an internal experience—the natural response to significant loss. And while dictionaries define grief as "a very great sadness" (Cambridge Dictionary, 2023a), grief is so much more than that. Grief is the natural reaction to significant loss *in totality* and includes physical, emotional, psychological, behavioral, social, and spiritual manifestations (Hall, 2014). In other words, sadness is just one component of the grief experience (See Table 1 for additional terminology, definitions, and distinctions).

*Table 1: Terminology and Definitions*

| Term | Definition |
|---|---|
| Death | The end of life, an irreversible cessation of biological functions required to sustain an organism. |
| Loss | Having less of, or no longer having, something that was cherished or with which there was an emotional bond. |
| Grief | Grief is the natural reaction to significant loss *in totality*, which includes physical, emotional, psychological, behavioral, social, and spiritual manifestations. |
| Grieving | The process of adjusting to life after significant loss. |
| Sadness | A specific emotional reaction to a specific event. It can cause temporary changes in mood or functioning but resolves on its own over a short or limited period. Daily functioning is not typically impacted. |
| Depres-sion | A mental illness featuring persistent feelings of sadness, worthlessness, and/or hopelessness that may or may not have a specific triggering event. It can significantly impair daily functioning and often requires professional treatment. |
| Bereave-ment | The process of adjusting to life after the death of a loved one. |
| Mourning | The culturally structured and externally facing response to grief. |

## Models of grief

Death, grief, and loss are historical constants in human life and how humans have coped with these inevitabilities has changed across time and across cultures (Jacobsen, 2021). The modern understanding of grief is that grief is a normal response to significant loss, not a disease in need of a cure. While older models of grief, as described below, frame grief as an obstacle to overcome or something a person needs to "move on" from, contemporary frameworks view grief as something a person keeps, and the work of healing is about making space for that grief rather than trying to get rid of it. The following discussion on the history of major grief models should be contextualized with the understanding that: 1) humans have managed and moved through grief and loss long before there were theoretical models; 2) there is no right or wrong way to grieve; and 3) that while these models are widely used in popular culture, they do not represent current understandings of grief.

Sigmund Freud is often credited with creating the first theoretical model on grief in his 1917 paper "MOURNING AND MELANCHOLIA" (Granek, 2010; Carhart-Harris et al., 2008; Harrer, 2018; Hall, 2014; McLean et al., 2022). Freud introduced the idea of "grief work," a series of tasks that had to be completed in sequential order for a person to "move on" from grief (Hall, 2014). Over the next 100 years, many more theorists would suggest models to explain the grief process. However, one model has dominated pop culture and public awareness (Stroebe et al., 2017; McLean et al., 2022), and that is the Kubler-Ross Model, colloquially known as the Five Stages of Grief (Kubler-Ross, 1969). This model, not unlike Freud's, views grief as something to be worked through via pre-determined tasks. Kubler-Ross formalized these tasks into five stages: denial, anger, bargaining, depression, and acceptance. These stages are distinct and each one is important to the healing process; failure to successfully complete any of the stages results in complications in recovering from grief (see Table 2 for descriptions of the five stages).

*Table 2: The Kubler-Ross Five Stages of Grief*

| Stage | Description |
|---|---|
| Denial | Conscious or unconscious refusal to acknowledge the reality of a situation; often a numbing of emotion |
| Anger | A stage of intense emotion after emerging from denial; expression of frustration, anger, or outrage at the situation, frequently including attempts to place blame |
| Bargaining | A process wherein a person attempts to distance themselves from their new reality or postpone it |
| Depression | Feelings of loneliness, despair, and helplessness in facing reality |
| Acceptance | Recognition or acknowledgement of reality and no longer attempting to deny, protest, or fight against it |

Given the popularity of this model, it's no surprise that the Kubler-Ross stages are frequently used when games integrate grief into their narratives, mechanics, and environments. For example, GRIS (Nomada Studio, 2018) is a wordless, visually stunning 2D platform-adventure game which uses the Kubler-Ross stages as a scaffold for level development and story progression (Sandra & Mutiaz, 2021; University of Cambridge, 2021). Similarly, the adventure-puzzle game RIME (Tequila Works,

2017) is narratively about loss and represents the five stages of grief as levels within an important in-game structure (Ahlgrim, 2018). From focusing on Denial in the indie title BEFORE YOUR EYES (GoodbyeWorld Games, 2021) to modeling Acceptance in Square Enix's NIER REPLICANT (Cavia, 2010), the five stages of grief has been and continues to be the major player in gaming's grief representations.

Unfortunately, as often happens when psychological research becomes integrated into pop culture, complex topics become flattened and oversimplified to the point where they are neither accurate nor helpful. This is the case for the Kubler-Ross model. The model dates to Kubler-Ross' 1969 book ON DEATH AND DYING, where she presented observations from interviews with hospitalized, terminally ill patients (Kubler-Ross, 1969). The model was groundbreaking in that it prioritized a patient-focused approach to death and gave voice to dying individuals who traditionally had been ignored (Stanford Medicine, 2019; Tyrrell et al., 2023). However, the model has been inappropriately applied to all people (not just those hospitalized with terminal conditions) and to all kinds of grief. Furthermore, the model's focus on orderly progression through neat and tidy stages has been widely criticized and rejected by mental health professionals (Stroebe et al., 2017; Corr, 2020; Hall, 2014). The model is also unhelpful to grieving individuals themselves (Maciejewski et al., 2007) and can even be actively harmful as it can cause grieving people to believe they are grieving incorrectly and thus negatively impact help-seeking from personal and professional support (Avis et al., 2021).

> "Stage theories put grieving people in conflict with their emotional reactions to losses that affect them. No matter how much people want to create simple, iron clad guidelines for the human emotions of grief, there are no stages of grief that fit every person or relationship." (Friedman & James, 2008; p. 41).

To be clear, this does not mean that games that integrate the whole or aspects of the Kubler-Ross model are harmful or inappropriate. Having clear, defined stages and progression fits neatly into how games are designed, and it makes complete sense that the model could be used in this way. The Kubler-Ross model can be helpful for those who see their experiences reflected in the model's stages, and those experiences are valid. However, there is so much more to grief and grieving than can be described by the rigid, predetermined progression offered by stage models. The goal of this work, therefore, is to encourage developers to move beyond the five stages and expand the portrayal of grief in games into places that are more empathic, humane, validating, and supportive. This is no small task. Although death, grief, and loss are universal, each instance is unique and deeply personal. Everyone grieves but no one grieves the same way. This is especially true when expanding the scope from individual grief to larger communal and cultural expressions and norms (Bregman, 2010).

> "No culture has ever been able to leave death to *itself* or just accept death *as it is* – all cultures have developed, for them, culturally specific ways of understanding and relating to this certainty of life. From historical epoch to epoch, from culture to culture, from one social group to another, from individual to individual, death is 'done' differently." (Jacobsen, 2021; p. 4)

## Why would we want these feelings in our games?

Grief comes in a variety of flavors, but is always rooted in the pain of losing. Games, on the other hand, are a space for joyful gaining. We enjoy games because most of the time we *gain* good feelings playing them. Whether crushing candies or slaying intergalactic space zombies, games are known for "fiero" moments, those epic wins that make you jump and cheer with victory. Where grief breeds distress, games can bring comfort and relaxation. Where grief leaves us feeling helpless or out of control, games can be empowering and enabling. Where grief drags us toward suffering, games push us to create and achieve the best versions of our idealized selves. And so, the question is: Why would anyone want grief in their games?

The answer lies in the connective tissue between grief and gameplay: emotion. Both games and grief make us feel things, often intensely and all at once. Emotions related to grief are often labeled as "bad" or "negative" (e.g. sadness, despair, lonely) while feelings experienced through gameplay are often considered "good" or "positive" (e.g. victorious, competent, connected). However, there are no "good" or "bad" feelings. While we do experience emotions on a spectrum from pleasant to unpleasant, all feelings are important and serve a purpose (Brackett, 2019). Sadness is just as valid and important a feeling as joy.

Many games, especially those that are routinely rated as "most meaningful," tap into the entire spectrum of human emotions, from pleasant and unpleasant (Jørgensen, 2016; Jørgensen, 2020). Losing a life or having a favorite character die is not a fun experience as it evokes a sense of loss. Humans often experience the fear of loss more intensely than the potential pleasure of gaining, a cognitive bias known as loss aversion. Loss in a game, however, can enhance opposite emotions when a player achieves a new high score or defeats the final boss. In other words, overcoming the challenge enhances a sense of victory or accomplishment.

It might sound ridiculous that video games, sometimes seen by general audiences as frivolous, silly fictional works, provide spaces for feeling emotions we typically avoid in our day-to-day lives. However, it is precisely because games are frivolous, silly, and fictional that we can observe, experience, and express a full range of human emotions. The freedom from reality, the freedom from consequence, and the freedom from productivity create a safe emotional space; death is not really death and loss is not really loss. This abstraction allows players to feel unpleasant emotions—but not too intensely—and to play with, stretch and subvert existentially terrifying concepts like death and experience gentler versions of overwhelming, though normal, emotional reactions like grief. In animal studies, play is often seen as a tool for preparing young critters with the skills and knowledge they'll need to survive in adulthood (Brown, 2010). So too can playing video games help prepare us for the universal experience that is loss.

## Games and the normalcy of death and loss

Death has been a part of video games since the beginning. Many of the earliest games, like SPACE INVADERS (Taito, 1978) and PAC-MAN (Namco, 1980), utilized the language of life and death to describe gameplay. For example, the term "lives" used to convey how many chances a player had before getting a "game over" screen. Modern games continue to use this language, and in many games, death is expected and often a stepping stone to success. For example, the roguelike genre is known for being exceedingly difficult, with players racking up dozens if not hundreds of deaths in their gameplay. In the pixel platformer CELESTE (Extremely OK Games, 2018), the player is expected to try, die, try again, die again, and eventually succeed. In fact, instead of having lives to lose, Celeste counts the number of player deaths and displays them like a badge of honor. These types of games embrace death as a sign of learning and growth.

Despite the frequency of death in games, the experience or depiction of grief is rare. Players may experience sadness at the death of a beloved NPC or frustration, anger, or despondency at having to restart a level or an entire game, but this is not the same as grief. The following is a specific examination of games that address grief in their gameplay and through the player experience.

## Games and grief

Games that address grief typically shed the frivolity of death and loss and embrace the power of difficult experiences and unpleasant consequences as part of meaning-making. For example, FIRE EMBLEM (Intelligent Systems, 1991) is a popular tactical RPG series famous for its "permadeath" mechanic. Permadeath refers to the permanent loss of a character in the game. When this happens, the player must either restart the entire mission or press on without the fallen ally. A modern example is UNDERTALE (Toby Fox, 2015), a 2D role-playing video game, which is designed to remind players that their actions have consequences. If the player defeats certain enemies and then resets the game, text will display something like "You have flashes of [character] dying". Should a player complete a "Genocide run" (a playthrough where the player kills every creature) and then attempt to complete a "Pacifist run" (every creature is spared), the gameplay changes and is reflective of the player's previous history of murder. Thus, there are consequences to actions and death carries an impact. However, these games are still short of evoking grief. Deconstructing these representations may help developers think about how these elements are being deployed and if the placement is right for the story they are trying to tell.

## Grief-adjacent games

Grief-adjacent games are those where grief and loss are not the focus but still play an important role in gameplay and the player experience. ANIMAL CROSSING: NEW LEAF (Nintendo, 2001) is a wonderful example of this. The cute, fun life simulator sees the player live alongside animal creatures as neighbors who often need favors or a helping hand. There is no death in this world: flowers can be stomped on, trees cut down, and the player can even be stung by bees, but there is no death. Despite the lack of death, the game can invoke powerful feelings of loss and grief. The animal neighbors who the player has come to befriend can move out and sometimes do so without a word. These NPCs can vanish without notice and leave behind nothing but a letter explaining their decision. The loss of a beloved digital critter is important even though it is not a death, and it can have an emotional impact on the player. The feeling is more than sadness; it is the feeling of absence and the reckoning of a world that is forever and irrevocably changed.

## Grief-centered games

Grief-centered games are games where grief and loss are core to the story, the mechanics, or the environment. Games such as LITTLE MISFORTUNE (Killmonday Games, 2019), ARISE: A SIMPLE TALE (Piccolo Studio, 2019), WHAT REMAINS OF EDITH FINCH (WROEF; Giant Sparrow, 2017), BROTHERS: A TALE OF TWO SONS (Starbreeze Studios, 2013), GRIS (Nomada Studio, 2018) and FINAL FANTASY VII all fit this bill. For example, the loss of controller functionality following the death of the older brother in BROTHERS: A TALE OF TWO SONS is a perfect example of how a game can mechanically represent loss. Not only does half the controller no longer work, but it *feels* odd to not have that control. That is, the loss is noticeable in a physical sense, which mirrors the physical discomfort, confusion, and emotional phantom limb-like sensation experienced during grief. In WROEF, the entire environment is one of peeling away layers of the unspeakable in search for meaning and understanding. GRIS, a beautifully crafted platformer, delivers a moving narrative without a single piece of dialog. The game slowly, artfully, and non-verbally reveals that the main character has lost her voice due to experiencing grief for her mother.

Games featuring strong themes of grief can be emotionally powerful. However, that power is somewhat mitigated by the directness, or lack thereof, of the grief theme. These types of games often skew more toward abstraction or artistic interpretation. They tend to rely heavily on symbolism or metaphor, which can grant players the distance needed to play and process heavy content without becoming overwhelmed—without having to look grief directly in the eye. They are a fantastic starting point for exploring grief and fostering meaningful conversations around death and loss; however, if games are going to truly change social norms and expectations around grief, loss, and death, more direct approaches need to be included in the catalog of grief games.

## Death-positive games

Lastly, there are games that are clearly and unequivocally about grief and loss and can be considered "death positive." The death positive movement contends that the culture of silence around death and dying is harmful and should be disrupted through, "discussion, gathering, art, innovation, and scholarship" (The Order of the Good Death, 2023). Therefore, death positive games are those that directly acknowledge the broader, more complex nature and impact of death, loss, and grief. Being death positive creates space for players to explore grief as a natural part of processing loss. THAT DRAGON, CANCER (Numinous Games, 2016), THE LAST CAMPFIRE (Hello Games, 2020), HOW TO SAY GOODBYE (Veltman et al., 2022), A MORTICIAN'S TALE (Laundry Bear Games, 2017), and SPIRITFARER (Thunder Lotus Games, 2020) are all examples of death-positive games. They defy taboo around discussing death and dying, normalize discussion of death and feelings of grief, and give voice and visibility to those in grief—a historically ignored perspective.

## Grief-game matrix

The following matrix is designed to give examples of how to consider grief presentation in games. Grief is complex and so too is representing it.

*Table 3: Grief-Game Matrix*

| **Grief Presentation Elements in Games** | | | |
|---|---|---|---|
| | Grief Adjacent | Grief Centered | Death Positive |
| Significant Loss | X | X | X |
| Loss Impacts Gameplay | X | X | X |
| Loss Causes Permanent Change | X | X | X |
| No attempt to "fix" the loss | | X | X |
| Normalizes grief and loss | | X | X |
| Unambiguous about grief and loss | | | X |
| Challenge social stigma | | | X |

At the top of the matrix are types of games that touch on grief to a varying extent. Grief-adjacent games are those that contain significant loss and that loss, though not a major game element, is both permanent and impacts gameplay. Grief-centered games meet the above criteria but take things a step further by having grief and loss at their core. The game is about grieving the loss of something or someone. These games don't attempt to "fix" or resolve the uncomfortable feelings of loss, but rather lean into discomfort through narrative, mechanical, and environmental means. Lastly, the death positive games are those that directly confront taboos around displaying the pain of grief and the discomfort of loss, incorporate frank yet humane discussion of death or loss, and challenge social stigmas that surround feeling and expressing grief. To provide additional insights into death positive games, below is an in-depth analysis of a quintessential example: A MORTICIAN'S TALE.

## *A Mortician's Tale.* A game that gets grief right

A MORTICIAN'S TALE has players take on the role of Charlie, aka Charlotte, a young woman recently hired by the local mom-and-pop funeral home Rose and Daughters. As a mortician, Charlie is responsible for managing the needs of both the living and the dead, from preparing bodies to reading emails. This duality of roles allows the game to address death, loss, and grief in two distinct ways: 1) the normalization of death as part of life; and 2) the critique of the death industry.

## Normalization of death

The core gameplay loop begins with the player receiving an email pertaining to an upcoming funeral service. The player gains additional information and insight by reading subsequent emails from the various cast. Once the administrative business is done, the player prepares the body for the upcoming service per the family's request. Preparations vary and can include burial, open/closed casket, or cremation. Once the body has been properly prepared, the game shifts focus from the dead to the living. Charlie changes into an all-black outfit and attends the funeral where the player pays their respects to the deceased and is encouraged to speak to the friends and family present at the service (See Figure 1). When one service ends, it's on to the next. Feelings of discomfort at attending the dead and the heaviness of mourning become less weighty as these tasks become routine. This isn't to say that each service doesn't carry emotional weight. The player is guided through simple yet purposeful actions, such as bathing a corpse, and these actions are repeated for each body, creating a rhythm to the gameplay loop. While these preparatory tasks can feel uncomfortable or even scary, there is an intimacy and comfort in going through these steps. The player is caring for these people prior to their final moments on this earth. Here at Rose and Daughters, death is a normal part of life.

*Figure 1: An example of Charlie at a funeral, speaking with attendees.*

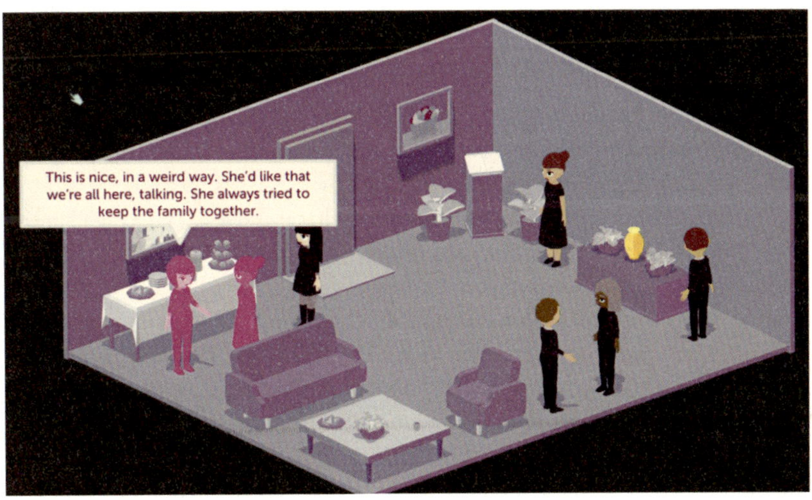
This is nice, in a weird way. She'd like that we're all here, talking. She always tried to keep the family together.

*Figure 2: Example of an email from Funerals Monthly*

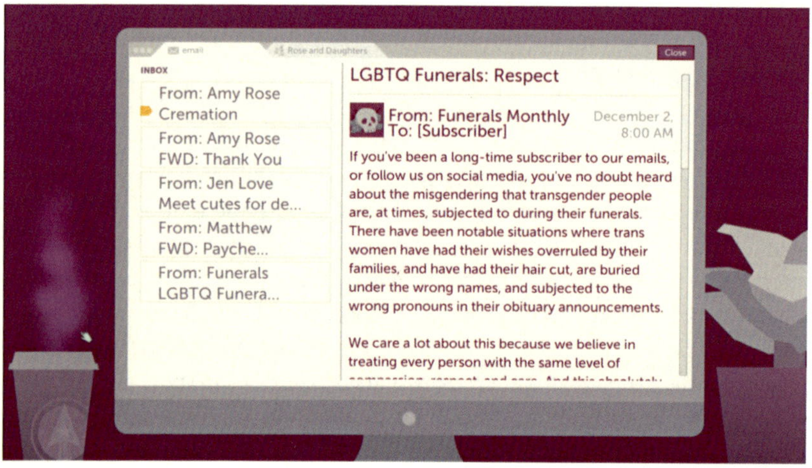


## The industry of death

A major plot point in A MORTICIAN'S TALE is the procedural rhetoric pertaining to the death industry that has thrived under a capitalistic society. Throughout the game, the player is provided information through emails and via overheard conversations about pressures for Rose and Daughters to be brought under new, more corporate-style management which immediately starts cutting corners, upselling users (which in this situation are people in mourning), and other profit-maximizing strategies. Death is unfortunately expensive. Transportation, preparation, coffins and urns, flowers, food, and staff wages all make dying financially costly. There are moments, such as when the new director excitedly highlights a pediatric contract with a local hospital as a boon for business, that leave a bitter taste in the mouth. While this relates specifically to monetary costs, environmental costs are also addressed in the game. Caskets and burials are typically not eco-friendly, and the energy used in a cremation is significant. One is left to wonder if there isn't another way.

These two facets tap into the real nature of what it is like to be engaged in the death process. Being involved with death and grief through this lens highlights the potentially extortive and manipulative nature of those seeking to profit from a devastating but natural occurrence. Alternatively, the game spotlights how vital people in this role are as they prepare the deceased for their final rest. Confronting the cold, hard facts of death directly contributes to a death-positive framing. As noted earlier, the game does not shy away from the emotional and physical challenges of death and grief, nor does it sensationalize it. This creates a grounding and engaging experience for the player. Ultimately, Charlie opens her own funeral parlor that abides by her own values of humane treatment and eco-consciousness.

Beyond the procedural rhetoric and social commentary, A MORTICIAN'S TALE does an excellent job of preserving the humanity of grief. It may sound odd out of context, but while the game approaches death and dying with the seriousness it deserves, it is not afraid to laugh. This tends to come from funeral guests in the form of adults remarking on the quality of the food or a child playing a video game during a wake. Emails from Jen (friend) and Matt (co-worker) also provide some excellent moments of humor. Jen suggests Charlie sign up for "Dead Meets," a dating website for death positive people: "Meet cutes for death positive cuties." Matt tells a tale of driving a hearse through a drive-thru and the ensuing confusion and hilarity of people's reactions. While some may think joking or making light of death is inappropriate, these examples highlight and reinforce that it is perfectly natural to feel something other than crushing sadness in the face of death. It also disrupts the common misconception that there is a "right way" to grieve; people experiencing grief may feel nothing or may want to laugh. Either response is appropriate, and it is the freedom to express those emotions, whatever they may be, that lends itself toward healing. By incorporating both in the game, the developers gave voice and representation to the normal, broad range of grief reactions. This shifts the focus from outright sadness and promotes a level of growth both for the player and Charlie on their journeys.

Another very common, very human reaction to grief is concerned with the social support system surrounding the aggrieved. Social support plays a significant part in achieving positive outcomes after a loss, such as decreased risk of suicide (Pitman et al., 2020) or developing depression (Fried et al., 2015) and increases the capacity for coping (Harrop et al., 2020). However, support for those in grief is often inadequate due to lack of education about or comfort with supporting someone in grief (Devine, 2017; Stroebe et al., 2017). We are not taught effective strategies for supporting people in grief, and people often feel at a loss for what to say and/or fear saying something wrong and making matters worse (Devine, 2017).

This is yet another situation where A MORTICIAN'S TALE shines. As a funeral director, the player is treated as a trusted person who understands bereavement and is provided opportunities to practice empathic, appropriate support. The game equips the player with grief psychoeducation around what to say through the gameplay itself. For example, the player receives updates from "Funerals Monthly," a newsletter for morticians, that provides transferable pieces of advice such as "What Not to Do at a Funeral," "Understanding Different Funeral Practices," "LGBTQIA+ Funerals," and "Avoid These Words" that can be helpful outside the game (See Figure 2).

In summary, A MORTICIAN'S TALE deals with death, dying, and grief in a way that is humane and realistic. It presents genuine and well-rounded portrayals of grief and loss and is designed to impart death positivity, or at least lessen fear and confusion around grief and loss. This game is not for everyone as there are experiences in A MORTICIAN'S TALE that may be too intense or distressing for some players. However, the game takes great strides in normalizing death, in showing the diverse range of ways grief is experienced and expressed, in educating players on how to support someone in grief, and in modeling the potential for games to destigmatize grief and loss (and not a stage in sight!).

## Grief game summary

All three of these types of grief games have a role to play in shifting social and cultural norms around death, loss, and grief. Grief-adjacent games help raise these topics, usually across wide swaths of game players. Grief-centered games allow players the opportunity to practice, in a safe way, the experience of grief and loss and can provide emotionally powerful moments of validation and normalization. Death-positive games take the experience afforded by grief-centered games and expands it from the individual to communal, and from personal to political. To challenge stigma, these games directly address grief events and the subsequent emotional processing. This directness may be off-putting or overwhelming for some players, and that's OK—every grief journey is different.

## Conclusion

Grief is the psychological, physical, emotional, social, and spiritual response to significant loss. Despite being one of the few universal human experiences, open discussion or expression of grief is considered taboo. Those in grief are encouraged or expected by society to hide their distress, and to "work through" their grief so that they can "move on." What little information is in the public consciousness around grief largely relates to the Kubler-Ross 5 Stages of Grief, a model that endorses a predictable and orderly progression through grief. However, the efficacy of this model has been rejected by modern grief researchers; everyone grieves differently and there is no right or wrong way to grieve.

To quote grief and games scholar Sabine Harper, "Video games are the medium of loss and death" (2018, p. 9) and, as the dominant media form of the 21st century, have the potential to shift social norms and destigmatize death, grief, and loss. Video games have embraced death and loss since the beginning and are no stranger to evoking intense emotional reactions. Many games are designed to elicit unpleasant feelings like sadness, confusion, or even helplessness, and yet players still play (and enjoy!) them. Research has even found that experiencing these unpleasant feelings, including grief, can play an important role in generating meaningful gameplay experiences.

This paper identified several grief-inclusive games and provided a simple matrix for understanding how different gameplay experiences can support and reinforce more accurate and humane understandings of grief and loss. While some of these games are artistic spaces for reflection and expression, others are direct dialogs on grief. Both experiences are critical to calling in players at a variety of different stages of grief education and understanding. Through discussion, education, modeling, and play, games can make the world a less stigmatizing, more informed, and more supportive place for those in grief.

## References


Ahlgrim, R. (2018, February). "Rime" tackles grief with puzzles. *Basement Medicine*.

Avis, K., Stroebe, M., & Schut, H. (2021). Stages of Grief Portrayed on the Internet: A Systematic Analysis and Critical Appraisal. *Frontiers in Psychology*, *12*. https://doi.org/doi: 10.3389/fpsyg.2021.772696

Brackett, M. (2019). *Permission to Feel: Unlocking the Power of Emotions to Help Our Kids, Ourselves, and Our Society Thrive*. Celadon Books.

Bregman, L. (2010). *Religion, death, and dying Volume 3: Bereavement and Death Rituals* (Lucy Bregman, Ed.). Praeger Publishers.

Brown, S. (2010). *Play: How it Shapes the Brain, Opens the Imagination, and Invigorates the Soul*. Avery.

Cambridge Dictionary. (2023a). *GRIEF | English meaning – Cambridge Dictionary*. Cambridge Dictionary Online. https://dictionary.cambridge.org/dictionary/english/grief?q=Grief

Cambridge Dictionary. (2023b). *LOSS | English meaning – Cambridge Dictionary*. Cambridge Dictionary Online. https://dictionary.cambridge.org/dictionary/english/loss

Carhart-Harris, R. L., Mayberg, H. S., Malizia, A. L., & Nutt, D. (2008). Mourning and melancholia revisited: correspondences between principles of Freudian metapsychology and empirical findings in neuropsychiatry. *Annals of General Psychiatry*, 7(1), 9. https://doi.org/10.1186/1744-859X-7-9

Cavia. (2010). NIER: REPLICANT. (Xbox 360 version). [Video game]. Square Enix.

Corr, C. (2020). Elisabeth Kübler-Ross and the Five Stages Model In Selected Social Work Textbooks. *Illness, Crisis, and Loss*, *30*(2). https://doi.org/10.1177/1054137320932302

Coward-Gibbs, M. (2020). *Death, Culture & Leisure×: Playing Dead* (in M. Coward-Gibbs, Ed.; 1st ed.). Emerald Publishing Limited.

Davis, J. (2022, April). The Importance of Seeing Grief Storylines on TV. *Harper's Bazaar*.

Devine, M. (2017). *It's OK That You're Not OK: Meeting Grief and Loss in a Culture That Doesn't Understand* (1st ed.). Sounds True.

Extremely OK Games. (2018). CELESTE. (Nintendo Switch Version). [Video game]. Extremely OK Games.

Florea, M.-L., & Rabatel, A. (2011). Media Representations of Death and the Issues Involved in the Construction of the Event. *Questions de communication* [En ligne], 20 | 2011, mis en ligne le 01 février 2014, consulté le 18 septembre 2023. http://journals.openedition.org/questionsdecommunication/8886

Fried, E. I., Bockting, C., Arjadi, R., Borsboom, D., Amshoff, M., Cramer, A. O. J., Epskamp, S., Tuerlinckx, F., Carr, D., & Stroebe, M. (2015). From loss to loneliness: The relationship between bereavement and depressive symptoms. *Journal of Abnormal Psychology, 124*(2), 256–265. https://doi.org/10.1037/abn0000028

Friedman, R., & James, J. (2008). The myth of the stages of dying, death, and grief. *Skeptic, 14*(2), 37–42.

Giant Sparrow. (2017). WHAT REMAINS OF EDITH FINCH. (PC Version). [Video game]. Annapurna Interactive.

GoodbyeWorld Games. (2021). BEFORE YOUR EYES. (PC version). [Video game]. Skybound Games.

Granek, L. (2010). Grief as pathology: The evolution of grief theory in psychology from Freud to the present. *History of Psychology, 13*(1), 46–73. https://doi.org/10.1037/a0016991

Hall, C. (2014). Bereavement theory: Recent developments in our understanding of grief and bereavement. *Bereavement Care, 33*(1), 7–12. https://doi.org/10.1080/02682621.2014.902610

Harper, Sabine. (2018). *Games and Bereavement.* Transcript Verlag.

Harrop, E., Scott, H., Sivell, S., Seddon, K., Fitzgibbon, J., Morgan, F., Pickett, S., Byrne, A., Nelson, A., & Longo, M. (2020). Coping and wellbeing in bereavement: Two core outcomes for evaluating bereavement support in palliative care. *BMC Palliative Care, 19*(1), 29. https://doi.org/10.1186/s12904-020-0532-4

Hello Games. (2020). THE LAST CAMPFIRE. (Nintendo Switch Version). [Video game]. Hello Games.

Intelligent Systems. (1991). FIRE EMBLEM. (Famicom Version). [Video game]. Nintendo.

Ivy, D. (2022). Grief as Taboo: Lewis, Burleson, and the Communication of Grief. In G. Luurs (Ed.), *Handbook of Research on Communication Strategies for Taboo Topics.* IGI Global. https://doi.org/10.4018/978-1-7998-9125-3

Jacobsen, M. (2021). Introduction: The whole world is watching – death in a spectacular age. In M. Jacobsen (Ed.), *The Age of Spectacular Death* (1st Edition, p. 1–19). Routledge.

Jacobsen, M., Lund, P., & Peterson, A. (2020). Spectacular Grief – On the individualisation, professionalisation and memorialisation of grief in contemporary society. In M. Jacobsen (Ed.), *The Age of Spectacular Death* (1st Edition, p. 161–183). Routledge.

James, J., & Friedman, R. (2017). Grief: A Neglected and Misunderstood Process. In *The Grief Recovery Handbook, 20th Anniversary Expanded Edition: The Action Program for Moving Beyond Death, Divorce, and Other Losses including Health, Career, and Faith* (20th Anniv, pp. 3–9). William Morrow Paperbacks.

Johnson, M. R. (2019). Inclusion and exclusion in the digital economy: Disability and mental health as a live streamer on Twitch.tv. *Information Communication and Society*, 22(4), 506–520. https://doi.org/10.1080/1369118X.2018.1476575

Jørgensen, K. (2016). The positive discomfort of Spec Ops: The Line. *The International Journal of Computer Game Research*, 16(2).

Jorgensen, K. (2020). When is it Enough? Uncomfortable Game Content and the Transgression of Player Taste. In K. Jorgensen & F. Karlsen (Eds.), *Transgression in Games and Play* (pp. 153–168). MIT Press.

Kahler, J., Papa, A., Epstein, E., & Levin, C. (2019). Attributions about bereaved spouses: Testing the myths of coping with loss. *Journal of Death and Dying*, 84(1), 307–334. https://doi.org/https://doi.org/10.1177/0030222819890974

Killmonday Games. (2019). LITTLE MISFORTUNE. (PC version). [Video game]. Killmonday Games.

Kubler-Ross, E. (1969). *On Death and Dying*. Macmillan.

Laundry Bear Games. (2017). A MORTICIAN'S TALE. (PC version). [Video game]. Laundry Bear Games.

Lund, P. (2022). Recreational grief as resonance – sociological notes on grief in popular culture. *Mortality*, 27(1), 90–106. https://doi.org/10.1080/13576275.2020.1823354

Maciejewski, P., Zhang, B., Block, S., & Prigerson, H. (2007). An empirical examination of the Stage Theory of Grief. *JAMA*, 297(7), 716–723. https://doi.org/doi:10.1001/jama.297.7.716

McLean, E., Singer, J., Laurita, E., Khaler, J., Levin, C., & Papa, A. (2022). Perception of grief responses: Are maladaptive grief responses and the stages of grief considered normal? *Death Studies*, 46(6), 1414–1423. https://doi.org/10.1080/07481187.2021.1983890

Merriam-Webster. (n.d.). *No Title*. Merriam-Webster.Com Dictionary. Retrieved September 15, 2023, from https://www.merriam-webster.com/dictionary/death

Morreall, J. (1968). Aristotle And the Paradox Of Tragedy. *The Angle*, 1.

Namco. (1980). PAC-MAN. (Arcade version). [Video game]. Midway.

Nintendo. (2001). ANIMAL CROSSING: NEW LEAF. (GameCube version). [Video game]. Nintendo.

Nomada Studio. (2018). GRIS. (PC Version). [Video game]. Devolver Digital.

Numinous Games. (2016). THAT DRAGON CANCER. (PC version). [Video game]. Numinous Games.

Piccolo Studio. (2019). ARISE: A SIMPLE TALE. (PC version). [Video game]. Untold Stories.

Pitman, A. L., King, M. B., Marston, L., & Osborn, D. P. J. (2020). The association of loneliness after sudden bereavement with risk of suicide attempt: a nationwide survey of bereaved adults. *Social Psychiatry and Psychiatric Epidemiology*, 55(8), 1081–1092. https://doi.org/10.1007/s00127-020-01921-w

Sandra, N., & Mutiaz, I. (2021). The embodiment of Kübler-Ross Model through game elements in GRIS and its impact on player experience. *The 2nd International Conference on Art, Craft, Culture, and Design*. https://www.atlantis-press.com/article/125967805.pdf

Stanford Medicine. (2019). *What the Elizabeth Kubler-Ross Archive Means to the Department of Medicine*. Department of Medicine: News. https://medicine.stanford.edu/news/current-news/standard-news/Kubler-Ross-Archive.html

Starbreeze Studios. (2013). BROTHERS: A TALE OF TWO SONS. (PC version). [Video game]. 505 Games.

Stroebe, M., Schut, H., & Boerner, K. (2017). Cautioning health-care professionals: Bereaved persons are misguided through the stages of grief. *Journal of Death and Dying*, 74(4). https://doi.org/10.1177/0030222281769187

Taito. (1978). SPACE INVADERS. (Arcade version). [Video game]. Taito.

Tequila Works. (2017). RIME. (Xbox One version). [Video game]. Grey Box.

The Order of the Good Death. (2023). *Death Positive Movement*. Accessed September 17, 2023. Retrieved from: https://www.orderofthegooddeath.com/death-positive-movement/

Thunder Lotus Games. (2020). SPIRITFARER. (PC version). [Video game]. Thunder Lotus Games.

Toby Fox. (2015). UNDERTALE. (PC version). [Video game]. Toby Fox.

Tyrrell, P., Harberger, S., Schoo, C., & Siddiqui, W. (2023). Kubler-Ross Stages of Dying and subsequent models of grief. *Stat Pearls*.

University of Cambridge. (2021). *Unspeakable: The Colour of Grief in Gris*. A Good Death. https://good-death.english.cam.ac.uk/reflections/unspeakable-the-colour-of-grief-in-gris/

Veltman, F., Portefaix, B., & ARTE France. (2022). HOW TO SAY GOODBYE. (PC version). [Video game]. ARTE France.

# The Strong Female Protagonist
## Stereotype Activation in Character Design and Its Psychological Impact

*Danielle Kelly and Bethany Thomas*

The video game industry had an estimated 3 billion players worldwide in 2022 (Statista, 2023) with 56% of those players estimated to be female (Statista, 2023). Despite this staggering statistic, gaming culture is perceived as being a predominantly male domain (Kelly et al., 2023). Historically, video games targeted male audiences (Cassel & Jenkins, 1998) perpetuating a long-standing gender hierarchy within gaming domains that is proving difficult to combat. An abundance of psychological research has explored gender inequality in gaming spaces to combat the hostility towards female players and increase female representation in games (e.g., Fox & Tang, 2017; Jagayat & Choma, 2021). A significant portion of the research has focused on the impact of hostility on players. However, it is also important to consider the responsibility of game companies and the toxic cultures they generate.

Gaming companies are responsible for promoting a culture that is accessible, representative and inclusive, yet their content often reflects and portrays exclusion and outdated stereotypes. For example, researchers have demonstrated the important relationship between game characters, avatars, and protagonists and the impact on player identity exploration and emotions (e.g., Yoon & Vargas, 2014; McMenomy, 2011; Kim et al., 2012; Hooi & Cho, 2014).

Such findings highlight the crucial role of characters in game content and their impact and potential benefits for players in the physical world. Despite this, negative portrayals of female players and femininity are perpetuated through lack of representation, gameplay, and character design. For example, female characters are typically portrayed as secondary, weak, or highly sexualized (Burgess et al., 2007; Downs & Smith, 2010; Summers & Miller, 2014; Lynch et al., 2016), and the roles of female characters have often been confined to caretakers, mothers, or love interests. Instances when female characters have opposed these portrayals are often followed by a backlash with misogynistic undertones, such as the response to the strong female character Abby in THE LAST OF US PART II (Naughty Dog, 2020) (Inverse, 2020). These portrayals are suggested to have a real-world negative impact on female players, normalizing sexual harassment (Dill et al., 2008; Yao et al., 2010), diminishing female players' self-efficacy (Behm-Morawitz & Mastro, 2009) and increasing their self-objectification (Fox et al., 2013; Vandenbosch et al., 2016).

These findings highlight the importance of understanding the role of gender stereotypes in gaming domains. The impact of gender representation through the portrayal of female characters on female players is incredibly complex. Crucially, the negative gender-based stereotypes portrayed by female characters are overwhelming and the negative gender-based stereotypes towards female players are similarly undisputable. The current chapter aims to discuss these in tandem, exploring the portrayal and design of female game characters, and the impact on female players. Throughout this chapter, we will draw on relevant theoretical underpinnings and literature from psychology, as they provide foundations for understanding the gender inequalities within the gaming domain, applying these to popular games as case studies, specifically TOMB RAIDER (Crystal Dynamics, 2013) and HORIZON ZERO DAWN (Guerilla Games, 2017).

## Stereotype Content Model

To combat the gender hierarchy in gaming, we first need to understand why it exists and some of the underlying psychological theories that support it. Buyukozturk (2022) suggests that the gender hierarchy that exists within gaming spaces is due to the gender inequality created in these domains. According to research from Buyukozturk (2022) women will "trade place for peace" (p. 1) in gaming contexts. The consistent harassment towards women in gaming spaces leads them to try to minimize their presence, while men will take this minimization as a lack of presence – awareness of the difference between these is crucial. Consequently, the lack of female presence further perpetuates gaming as male-dominated, where non-male players are perceived as subordinate or 'other'. The justification of male dominance is further supported by the overwhelming lack of representation within digital spaces. As discussed, females are underrepresented in digital game content, with the limited existing representations often adhering to negative stereotypes. These stereotypes, according to social psychological literature, tend to be generated according to two main dimensions: the perceived warmth and competence of the social group (Fiske et al., 2002).

The dimensions of warmth and competence form the foundations of what is known as the Stereotype Content Model. According to this model (Fiske et al., 2002), we elicit feelings towards others depending on how we perceive these dimensions. Fiske and colleagues' model suggests that there are various traits we measure the components of warmth and competence on when creating a perception of someone. Warm traits tend to include being good-natured, trustworthy, tolerant, and sincere, while competent traits include being capable, skillful, intelligent, and confident. The dimensions of warmth and competence incorporate existing traits present in other models. For example, Wojciske (2005) highlighted the traits of morality and competence in developing stereotypical perceptions. In comparison to warmth, the component of morality included other traits, such as being righteous and helpful. Consider these traits and their applications to game characters, a skillful and intelligent protagonist often portrayed through male characters, versus a good-natured and tolerant secondary character, the role of a caretaker often portrayed by a female character.

The combination of warmth and competence, in addition to components of morality, leads to the elicitation of certain emotions towards groups of people. For example, groups that are perceived to be low in both competence and warmth (Fiske uses the examples of the poor and the homeless here) will be met with feelings of disgust and contempt. Groups that are perceived to be high in both these dimensions are met with feelings of pride and admiration, such as citizens and those in the middle class (Fiske, 2018). More specific to gender stereotypes, women are rarely at the uniform ends of the warmth-competence model. Rather than being viewed as uniformly negative (low in warmth and competence) or uniformly positive (high in warmth and competence), women tend to be viewed as high in only one of the dimensions at a time (high in competence, low in warmth, or vice versa). As a result, women tend to be "respected or liked, but not both" (Connor & Fiske, 2018, p. 6) – once again, we can consider the backlash to the 'ability' of the character Abby (THE LAST OF US PART II) who kills Joel, a man—who happens to be the protagonist of the first entry in the series. The perception of groups in terms of warmth and competence indicates intent and behavior towards them.

Considering attitudes towards gender more specifically, sexism tends to communicate how women are perceived by men (Ramos et al., 2016). There are two primary types of sexism that communicate specific attitudes towards women: *hostile sexism* and *benevolent sexism*. Perhaps the less subtle of the two, hostile sexism reflects a generally antagonistic predisposition towards women who are perceived to be challenging the status quo (i.e., taking on non-traditional or masculine roles). In comparison, benevolent sexism consists of acclaim for women who take on "traditionally female roles" (Ramos et al., 2016) – the roles often portrayed in game characters: caretakers, mothers, and love interests. These types of sexism comprise their own sub-components and attitudes, including attitudes towards heterosexuality, paternalism and gender differentiation (Allen, 2023). Hostile sexism incorporates the sub-components of *heterosexual hostility*, in which men have a desire to dominate women. *Competitive Gender Differentiation* is also incorporated under hostile sexism, which refers to men viewing women as weak or less competent to help increase their social status. Finally, the component of hostile sexism also includes *dominant paternalism*, referring to the desired power dynamic between men and women.

In comparison, the sub-components of benevolent sexism display a different perspective. These sub-components include *heterosexual intimacy*, *complementary gender differentiation*, and *protective paternalism* (Glick et al., 2000). Heterosexual intimacy suggests that women are only viewed in terms of acting as necessary partners for men. Their main role is to support males, and much like the assigned roles of female characters in games, they are a secondary supporting character. Gender differentiation focuses more specifically on attributes; that is, there are particular "desirable traits" for women, such as purity. The final sub-component, protective paternalism, focuses on the belief that men are more powerful and competent than women, and are therefore charged with protecting them. Despite the different strengths of attitudes that can be seen in hostile and benevolent sexism, both share a common component. In terms of the warmth-competence model, both of these types of sexism indicate a belief that women are less competent than men which is a frequent stereotype female players currently face in gaming spaces, as evidenced by psychological research (e.g., Kaye et al., 2017; Gestos et al., 2018; Kelly et al., 2023).

## Stereotype activation and objectification theory

So what factors influence our perspective of the traits in the Stereotype Content Model? The activation of these stereotypes can happen through various methods, including objectification (Heflick et al., 2011).

Objectification refers to the act of viewing a human being as an object and, as a result, perceiving them as less than human (Heflick et al., 2011). It can be heavily influenced by encouraging someone to focus on someone else's appearance, particularly about females (Heflick & Goldenberg, 2009). Objectification Theory, in this respect, suggests that the sociocultural environment that we currently live in encourages the evaluation and objectification of women's bodies (Frederickson & Roberts, 1997). More specifically, the theory stipulates that women are taught to internalize this objectification and, in so doing, create the primary perspective of themselves from an outsider's view. The objectification of women plays a significant role in perceived judgments of warmth and competence. Heflick and Goldenberg (2009) found that, when asked to focus on a woman's appearance, the women were perceived as less competent. This raises an interesting conundrum when considering warmth and competence in the world of gaming. Whilst the characters in games are not 'real' humans, there is still a significant focus on how female characters look in these games, with clear attempts to encourage objectification with hypersexualized outfits or disproportional body types. Such sexualization impacts female players, as evidenced in the increasing stereotype of hypersexualized 'gamer girls', fueling negative gender-based stereotypes (Paaßen et al., 2017).

The objectification of female players, and game characters, is particularly crucial when we consider the long-standing archetypes of female characters in games.

## The archetype of the female game character

The characterization of female game characters reflects just some problematic attitudes when considered in conjunction with the theoretical frameworks discussed above. Female protagonists have been developed as weaker reflections of their male counterparts, portrayed as secondary characters or highly sexualized (Downs & Smith, 2010; Lynch et al., 2016). Their roles have often been confined to caretakers, mothers, or love interests, or, perhaps the most distressing of all archetypes, the sex object. Games have portrayed female characters in hypersexualized forms for decades, with limited consideration given to the development of these characters and the problematic out-of-game stereotypes these characters perpetuate.

Alarmingly, the sexualization of these characters and perpetuation of female characters as sex objects has been done, in some instances, intentionally. The hypersexualization of female characters by developers played a key role in catering to their perceived main demographic, males (Mikula, 2003). Although there has been a decrease in hypersexualized characters since 2006 (Anupama & Chithra, 2022), many games are still depicting key female characters as overly sexualized. Anupama and Chithra highlight the presence of Catwoman (Selina Kyle) in the BATMAN: ARKHAM game series (2009–2015). Despite her key role in progressing the game, there is a significant focus drawn to her body and movements, highlighted as being "seductive in nature" (Anupama & Chithra, 2022).

The design of hypersexualized characters is deliberate, created by gaming companies to fuel masculine power fantasies and, as a result, women do not tend to have major roles in the narrative (King & Douai, 2014). Even in instances when female characters are not necessarily designed as sexual objects, they can often be placed in subservient or secondary roles, such as the role of the *damsel in distress* (Maity, 2014; Summers & Miller, 2014). The damsel in distress often has a purpose in the narrative but rarely gets the opportunity to develop as a character. Rather, their main role is to create a situation for a male character to demonstrate their prowess as a protector. A prevalent example of this archetype can be found in the world of SUPER MARIO (Salter & Blodgett, 2017). Many of the games in the SUPER MARIO series have been focused on saving Princess Peach after she has been kidnapped, repeatedly, by Bowser. Despite the numerous variations of the Mario games, many of them have been designed around this exact premise.

Princess Peach's portrayal as a damsel in distress is not a unique situation. One of the more extreme presentations of this archetype can be found in RESIDENT EVIL 4 (Capcom, 2005), with the introduction of the president's daughter, Ashley Graham.

Ashley's introduction to the game became a point of contention for many fans. Not only was she consistently being kidnapped, but also often needed help with basic tasks such as getting down ladders. While the latter issue can be pinned down to game mechanics, her penchant for being kidnapped did not endear her to fans.

Ashley and Princess Peach's portrayals in these games are reminiscent of the stereotypes often encouraged by the protective paternalism aspect of benevolent sexism. While the concept of protective paternalism can seem generally positive in these situations, these feelings are elicited under the assumption that women are less competent than their male counterparts, and so require unsolicited help (Glick & Fiske, 1997). As demonstrated, this stereotype is one we frequently see impacting female players, as they are consistently perceived as less competent than male players (Kaye et al., 2017; Gestos et al., 2018; Kelly et al., 2023) and many female character designs continue to perpetuate this stereotype. Crucially, stereotype threats like this have been suggested to negatively affect task performance and prompt withdrawal from the associated domains; diminishing an individual's perception of their abilities, self-belief (Spencer et al., 2016) and interest in the task (Smith et al., 2007).

While creating situations that develop these paternalistic emotions towards the characters may seem harmless in comparison to the more hostile sexist depictions of females, unfortunately, the presence of any sexist representations in games can have a significant impact on how players behave in the outside world. Stermer and Burkley (2012) found that when men engaged with video games that could be perceived as sexist, they scored higher on measures of benevolent sexism than men who did not play these games. However, Stermer and Burkley (2012) identified a correlational relationship, rather than one of causation. In comparison, La Croix and colleagues (2018) experimentally manipulated the sex and sexuality of opponents in a first-person shooter and found that participants reported greater hostile sexism when their opponent was perceived as a sexualized female. Current research has also argued that female characters portraying and upholding negative gender-based stereotypes may have serious, real-world implications, as they normalize sexual harassment (Dill et al., 2008; Yao et al., 2010), diminish female players' self-efficacy (Behm-Morawitz & Mastro, 2009) and increase their self-objectification (Fox et al., 2013; Vandenbosch et al., 2017). Thus, the design of female characters as a means of perpetuating gender-based stereotypes, whether intentional or unintentional, can have a real-world impact on female players.

Critically, the removal of sexist portrayals in video games is not something that can be addressed in one singular manner. As highlighted above, numerous factors can demonstrate negative stereotypes of female characters. Firstly, many game developers rely on unrealistic body standards to create hypersexualized versions of women, designed to appeal to the perceived male demographic. Secondly, the lack of engagement with character development beyond using women as a secondary plot device in a traditionally female role prevents any movement away from established stereotypes and parallels the existing benevolent sexist tropes that exist in the physical world. There is, however, hope for the development of female characters out of the existing stereotypical frameworks. Some developers have been working to create fully fledged characters, both by recreating existing female protagonists (such as Lara Croft) and developing new protagonists that demonstrate how female characters can be depicted, discounting 'traditional' gender roles, bodies and narratives.

## The rise of *Tomb Raider*

The original TOMB RAIDER was released in 1996 by the developers Core Design and was published by Eidos Interactive. Lara Croft was designed as an archaeologist/adventurer, who is hired to acquire an artifact. Trouble ensues, with numerous other treasure hunters and interested parties also searching for the artifact. The game integrated elements of various genres, including gunfights, puzzles, and platforming. The games also used the novel third-person perspective throughout, providing significant excitement for its release. The historic introduction of Lara Croft in the TOMB RAIDER series opened the door for a new generation of female players, and the development of more fully formed female protagonists. Despite the introduction of Lara Croft as this strong female protagonist, however, the character was still significantly sexualized. As Du Preez (2007) highlights, the design of Lara Croft was mainly targeted at a core audience: teenage boys.

First, let us take a look at the original TOMB RAIDER (1996) and, in particular, Lara Croft's character design. The use of the third-person perspective in TOMB RAIDER provided the developers with an opportunity. In comparison to the first-person perspective, the third person allows you to see the avatar's full body. In the case of the Tomb Raider series, the angled third-person perspective lets the player view Lara Croft from behind – giving a visual fragmentation of Lara's Barbie-like proportions.

> "The visual clues supplied by Lara provide ample explanation for her popularity. Leggy Lara is usually clad in very short shorts, with clinging tops and boots to kick ass. She is also armed with a gun, knife and harpoon lately and is more than ready for action. The fact that Lara is top-heavy, to say the least...would make Dolly Parton, Pamela Anderson and old Barbie envious. Add to that her superhuman agility and no-nonsense sex appeal and you have a winner" (Du Preez, 2007, pp. 19–20).

The above quote was how Du Preez (2007) characterized the original Lara Croft, an idealized version of the female form. Lara Croft was originally designed to be a contradiction in terms; an overly sexualized female, with the ability to engage in typically 'masculine' pursuits, such as fighting, rock climbing, and riding a motorcycle. Du Preez also highlights that, what would normally be seen as a subversion of traditional female gender roles, was again a ploy by the developers to engage their typically male audience.

Some researchers have argued that the inclusion of both aspects of Lara Croft (her sexualization and competence in masculine traits) makes her neither a sex object nor a "feminist icon" (Engelbrecht, 2020). Looking at this from the perspective of the stereotype content model, however, the contradiction in terms may still cause figures such as Lara Croft to be perceived negatively. Despite her competence in particularly masculine traits, the sexualization of Lara Croft will cause players to target her appearance and, in doing so, encourage reduced perceptions of competence (Heflick & Goldberg, 2009). The focus on appearance could also be strengthened by the limited background in the first set of games. The player is placed in the game with limited contextual information provided on the character. This may have been deliberate; a lack of complexity to the character's personality provides a more simplified path to the creation of the "ideal female", highlighted by Du Preez (2007) as one of the aims of the developers.

The sexualization of Lara Croft seemed to form a significant part of player engagement with the game, so much so that some TOMB RAIDER players seemed to focus explicitly on Lara's appearance and the sexualized aspects of her form. The development of the Nude Raider patches provides evidence of this focus. These patches were a pornographic add-on that allowed players to remove Lara's clothing (BBC News, 1999). In doing so, perceptions of Lara as any kind of competent protagonist are removed – the patch allows players to only identify Lara as a fetishized character. This strengthens objectification, further dehumanizing Lara and encouraging a more hostile sexist view of her role in the game. When exploring this through the lens of objectification theory, the dehumanization of Lara Croft negates any attempts to increase perceptions of her competence. Whilst considering how this translates into the physical world, female players experiencing this are likely to internalize the objectification, creating an internalized perspective of themselves as less competent.

The consistent sexualization of Lara Croft did not improve in the sequels to the original game. In TOMB RAIDERS 2 and 3, the designers seemed to fixate on the sexualization of the character rather than focusing on the development of Lara Croft as a human or changing the environment to create further scope for interaction. Instead, the designers focused on changes to Lara's physique. The proportions of Lara's body became less realistic and more "obnoxiously sexualized" (LARA CROFT TOMB RAIDER series, 2001, as cited in Mikula, 2003). The lingering effects of the original TOMB RAIDER series created a ripple effect within the franchise reboot in 2013 and the rise of the TOMB RAIDER series, and the new games with new designs are an ideal comparison for the impact of each depiction of Lara. The reboot focuses on an earlier point of Lara's life – she has just become an archaeology graduate. At the start of an expedition, Lara finds herself stranded on an island after her ship is sunk in a violent storm and must develop hunting, combat and survival skills to survive the dangers of the island and complete her expedition.

The franchise reboot in 2013 deliberately redesigned Lara to be a stronger character with a more developed backstory. The complexity of Lara's character is evident from the start of the game. Lara's origin story creates a more complex overview of her development. At the start of the game, Lara is responsible for the ship steering into a dangerous area against another character's advice, after which point the ship gets damaged due to the storm. Her initial engagement in hunting and combat does not clearly demonstrate competence in these areas.

However, this deliberate mechanic that allows Lara's skills to develop in front of the player provides clearer cues for competence; there is a clear demonstration of skill development, leading to being skillful in dangerous situations. The inclusion of a skill tree provides further evidence for Lara's competence, demonstrating an increase in confidence and capability.

The complexity of Lara's development is not just evident in her growing competence. More in-depth interactions with other NPCs provide more social cues for individuals to positively interpret traits of warmth. Various interactions paint Lara as trustworthy and moral, as she fights to save her friends from various situations. Engelbrecht (2020) also highlights that the morphology facial technology used to create Lara's facial expressions was generated by an actress, and then imported into the game. Engelbrecht suggests that, as a result, this makes it more difficult to dehumanize and objectify the new Lara in comparison to the older two-dimensional version.

Perhaps one of the clearer progressions of Lara's character is her change in physique. Engelbrecht (2020) argues that Lara is no longer presented as a hypersexualized character. Rather, her physique is now more representative of an athletic woman, with no clear fixation on creating an idealized version of the female form (Macallum-Stewart, 2014). Engelbrecht also highlights that the clothing now worn by Lara are still figure-hugging, but no longer with the aim of sexualizing Lara's figure (Engelbrecht, 2020). The practicality of the clothing now worn by Lara should also be noted. The tight fit of the clothes aside, the 'short shorts' that the original Lara Croft first wore now have been replaced with trousers and boots – a more practical and realistic choice in the displayed environment.

One interesting factor to note about the TOMB RAIDER reboot is the presence of previous archetypes, namely the damsel in distress (Engelbrecht, 2020). Lara's friend Sam (short for Samantha) is kidnapped by inhabitants of the island, as they believe she could act as a successor to one of their deities. In comparison to the previous iterations of the archetype, however, Sam's role was not purely one of creating situations for a man to demonstrate his prowess over his female counterparts. Rather, Sam had a key role in the narrative of the story, creating clear, complex motivations both for Lara and the behavior of the island inhabitants. The role of Lara as the protagonist who 'saves the damsel in distress' is another subversion of traditional gender roles in gaming and seems to eliminate the presence of protective paternalism from the typical dynamic seen here. It should also be noted that it is unclear whether the inclusion of this type of archetype, even with a female protagonist, would elicit the same feelings of protective paternalism in the players, creating illusions of females as lacking competence. Regardless of how we interpret the use of the 'damsel in distress' archetype here, there can be limited argument that the redesign of Lara Croft in TOMB RAIDER influenced a new generation of female protagonists in the gaming world, one of the most influential being Aloy from HORIZON ZERO DAWN.

## *Horizon Zero Dawn*

HORIZON ZERO DAWN follows the story of Aloy, a hunter who must make her way through a post-apocalyptic world whilst hunting robotic creatures. Similar to the redesign of TOMB RAIDER, HORIZON ZERO DAWN had purposeful design elements that promoted female strength, moving away from the stereotypical archetypes of female characters in previous games. And crucial is the design of the female protagonist Aloy. In comparison to the world of TOMB RAIDER, however, the post-apocalyptic world that Aloy lives in goes further than just combating negative stereotypes associated with the protagonist. Various elements of the game were designed in a way that highlighted female characters in opposition to the societal traditional gender roles and characteristics that have been ascribed to femininity, including the game narrative and environment.

Aloy's narrative forms a key part of disrupting the female protagonist archetypes seen in historical games. Her journey begins as a child, with other children throwing stones at her due to her outcast status. Aloy's mentor, Rost, has been tasked with raising her by the Nora (a matriarchal tribe within the game) with the instruction to "raise it, not love it" (Guerilla Games, 2017 as cited in Allen, 2024). The statement here becomes key on two levels; the first is Rost's relationship with Aloy. Rost is protective of Aloy as a child but also provides her with the key skills she needs to complete her mission and survive (Allen, 2024).

This is reflective of the development we see in the early stages of TOMB RAIDER (2013), encouraging the player to focus consciously on the development of skills we would typically associate as masculine, and encouraging perceptions of competence.

The statement "raise it, not love it" provides an interesting perspective on the matriarchal Nora tribe. While HORIZON ZERO DAWN'S environment conflicts with typical action games that could typically be viewed as male-oriented, with a strong basis on hunting and combat, the game transposed these often male-oriented roles onto its female characters. The Nora seem to contradict the perceptions of traditional matriarchies. Matriarchal structures are often seen to demonstrate more "warm" traits, focusing on the women as caretakers or mothers (Goettner-Abendroth, 2018). The original statement about raising Aloy rather than loving her seems to be in direct conflict with what would typically be perceived as female traits. In comparison, in HORIZON these warm traits are treated as secondary to their hunting and combat skills.

The fact that the Nora are a matriarchy does not draw much focus within the game, which also reflects the focus on Aloy as a female. Remarkably, Aloy's gender is rarely used as an identifying characteristic, with the game preferring to focus on her status as an outsider (Allen, 2023). Allen highlights that, because of this focus, typical gender norms are not applied, opening the possibilities that Aloy's character has. The same logic can be applied to Aloy's relationships. The character almost avoids romantic entanglements throughout the game, preferring instead to focus on the task at hand. The lack of male figures discourages any kind of engagement with heterosexual intimacy, avoiding the influx of benevolent sexism. Aloy also has strong relationships with her friends, which helps develop the story as the game moves forward.

The focus on friendships over romantic relationships, as highlighted by Allen (2024), demonstrates that the romantic heteronormative relationships we normally see in games with a female protagonist are not necessary for the narrative. Instead, friendships can provide a similar level of complexity and emotional engagement.

The relationships highlighted in HORIZON ZERO DAWN are not the only factors that contradict typical constructs that encourage sexist beliefs. Aloy's presentation within the game completely removes many of the factors that could encourage the objectification of the main protagonist. From the first presentation of Aloy, she is dressed in hunter's garb, designed to live in her environment. The clothes she wears are not form-fitting, but rather provide armor and protection against the elements. Aloy's body proportions are not overly sexualized or overly feminine, and because her clothing reflects similar shapes and styling to the rest of the tribe, there are limited cues that would cause the player to target her appearance, reducing the likelihood of Aloy being objectified and reducing stereotypical activation.

The presentation of Aloy as a complex character has significant implications for representations of females both in the digital world and in the physical world. As with Lara Croft's redesign, Aloy's design removes the likelihood of dehumanization and objectification. As a result, women in the physical world are less likely to internalize these perspectives, promoting higher self-belief, particularly within the dimensions of competence.

Interestingly, however, the reaction to these changes in female protagonists is not always met with positive feedback. Concerning both TOMB RAIDER and HORIZON ZERO DAWN, literature has highlighted negative reactions to the removal of objectifying female features (e.g., see Allen, 2024). Some players argued that

Aloy's new "frame" was too masculine, removing the apparent "necessary" feminine curves that make her identifiably female (Nightingale, 2021). Statements such as these raise questions regarding the removal of 'traditional' femininity to combat negative stereotypes, when in fact it is the initial/inherent sexual objectification of femininity that is a problem. This further highlights the complex relationship between the world of gaming and real-world attitudes. The use of game design to reduce negative stereotypes can have far-reaching consequences, as highlighted by the negativity depicted by those who still hold sexist beliefs.

## Discussion and recommendations

When stereotype reduction in gaming is discussed, it is often talked about purely from the perspective of how the female characters are designed from a body proportion and clothing perspective. As highlighted in both TOMB RAIDER and HORIZON ZERO DAWN, these are both key components of reducing negative stereotypes. By encouraging the design of female protagonists with realistic body proportions and realistic clothing, we can reduce the objectification of these characters and, in turn, reduce engagement with factors that can encourage negative stereotype activation. Some factors of game design that are now possible can help implement assets that reduce negative stereotypes. As highlighted by Engelbrecht (2020), the use of morphology technology in more modern games provides an opportunity to create characters with more realistic facial expressions and encourage further identification with them and reduce objectification.

However, as we have also discussed, reducing gender-based negative stereotypes cannot be combated simply by changing a character's body type – the narrative and environment the female protagonists are placed in are also important. If we revisit the SCM at this point, we are reminded that women are often perceived as either warm or competent, but rarely both – leading to increased prejudicial beliefs (Connor & Fiske, 2018). By encouraging females to be characterized as both warm and competent, positive reactions towards women more generally can be elicited. In both the cases of the new Lara Croft and Aloy, we can see the development of both competence and warmth – a combination rarely seen in female video game protagonists.

In the case of Aloy, there is a subversion of typical female characteristics. Her exceptional skill with various weapons highlights a significant level of competence, particularly when compared to male NPCs within the game (Allen, 2024). However, Aloy also demonstrates traits we would associate with characteristics of warmth, so much so that players are at times given the choice to react to a scenario using various options, including compassion (a key indicator of warmth), strategy, or physicality. Allen (2024) argues that there seems to be a preference for making Aloy react in a compassionate way, reflecting the stereotypical expectations of how a woman should react in these situations. However, this can also reflect the complexity of Aloy as a character. Warmth is often not attributed to women whenever they are in domains that could be traditionally described as masculine, such as the environment Aloy is placed in (Kelly et al., 2023). However, the decision to engage with the compassionate response in this environment provides the opportunity for Aloy to demonstrate not only characteristics of competence, but also characteristics of warmth in an unexpected domain.

By the end of both TOMB RAIDER and HORIZON ZERO DAWN, Aloy and Lara Croft can be described as exceedingly competent. Allen (2024) highlights that, in the case of Aloy, some call her a *Mary Sue,* the term used to describe female characters when they have abilities that are unexplainable. However, with both TOMB RAIDER and HORIZON ZERO DAWN, there is a complexity to the gameplay that helps players become consciously aware of their protagonists' growing competence, removing any unexplained aspect of their abilities. In the case of Aloy, we see how Rost helped her develop her skills throughout her childhood. In comparison, we see Lara Croft start to understand her own abilities and develop skills through a baptism of fire in TOMB RAIDER. Like Aloy, Lara also manages to demonstrate compassion for her friends and colleagues in very masculine domains, providing clear indicators of warmth whilst maintaining her competence. The combination of both components highlights the complexity of the relationship between how a character is presented and the overall narrative of the story. Aspects of warmth and competence need to be carefully balanced to develop female characters that truly subvert traditional gender norms.

We do have to be aware, however, that even if a female protagonist is competent and warm, presenting them in an oversexualized way can counteract these positive perceptions. The presentation of the female protagonist is also not the only aspect of the game that can assist with the reduction of negative stereotypes. Comparatively, placing a female protagonist in the role of damsel in distress is likely to encourage feelings of protective paternalism and increase the likelihood of negative stereotype activation, regardless of how the female character is presented.

To focus purely on the role of the female protagonist would also be counterproductive. The position of other female characters within the game environment, such as Sam's role in TOMB RAIDER and the Nora in HORIZON ZERO DAWN, provide the opportunity for subversion of gender roles on a larger scale and provide further representation throughout the gaming world. This also extends to the relationships that the protagonists have with other characters. Heterosexual relationships between female protagonists and NPCs need to be carefully cultivated to ensure that the dynamic does not encourage benevolent sexism, particularly heterosexual intimacy.

Overall, game design can have a significant impact on perpetuating negative gender-based stereotypes and thus equally has an important role in the reduction of negative stereotypes. However, there is a complex balance to be struck between the presentation of the character, the narrative, and the environment. Both the reimagining of Lara Croft and the design of HORIZON ZERO DAWN demonstrate how key elements of game design can help counteract the negative stereotypes we have historically seen cultivated in games. By using the character design elements discussed here as the foundations of building complex female characters, games have a profound potential to continue building positive representations of women in the gaming domain, in turn having a positive psychological impact on female players and creating a more inclusive gaming culture.

## References

Aghazadeh, S. A., Burns, A., Chu, J., Feigenblatt, H., Laribee, E., Maynard, L., Meyers, M., O'Brien, J.L., & Rufus, L. (2018). GamerGate: A Case Study in Online Harassment. *Online Harassment*, 179–207.

Allen, M. L. (2024). "How is it that Someone Like You: Paragon, Damn Near Saint; Could Love this World so Damn Much but No One in It?": Horizon Zero Dawn's Aloy and the Disruption of Hetero-Amatonormative Benevolent Sexism in Female-led Games. *Games and Culture*, 15554120231179511.

Anupama, K., & Chithra, G. K. (2022). Of Castration Anxiety and Hypersexualized Female Bodies: A Critical Assessment of the Objectifying Gaze in Batman: Arkham Video Game Series. *Theory and Practice in Language Studies*, 12(9), 1921–1929. https://doi.org/10.17507/tpls.1209.26

BBC News (1999, March 18). Sci/Tech'Nude Raiders' face legal action. *BBC*. Retrieved 29/9/23:http://news.bbc.co.uk/1/hi/sci/tech/299040.stm

Behm-Morawitz, E., & Mastro, D. (2009). The effects of the sexualization of female video game characters on gender stereotyping and female self-concept. *Sex Roles* 61, 808–823. https://doi.org/10.1007/s11199-009-9683-8

Buyukozturk, B. (2022). Reproducing the gaming gender hierarchy. *Symbolic Interaction*, 45(1), 27–49. https://doi.org/10.1002/symb.553

Cassell, J., & Jenkins, H. (Eds.). (2000). *From Barbie® to Mortal Kombat: Gender and Computer Games*. MIT press.

Connor, R. A., & Fiske, S. T. (2018). Warmth and competence: A feminist look at power and negotiation. In C. Travis & J. W. White (Eds.). *APA Handbook of the Psychology of Women: History, Theory, and Battlegrounds*. American Psychological Association. https://doi.org/10.1037/0000059-000

Dill, K. E., Brown, B. P., & Collins, M. A. (2008). Effects of exposure to sex-stereotyped video game characters on tolerance of sexual harassment. *Journal of Experimental Social Psychology* 44(5), 1402–1408. https://doi.org/10.1016/j.jesp.2008.06.002

Downs, E., & Smith, S. L. (2010). Keeping abreast of hypersexuality: A video game character content analysis. *Sex roles* 62, 721–733. https://doi.org/10.1007/s11199-009-9637-1

Du Preez (2000). Virtual Babes: Gender, Archetypes and Computer Games. *Communication* 26(2), 18–27, DOI: 10.1080/02500160008537909

Engelbrecht, J. (2020). The New Lara Phenomenon: A Postfeminist Analysis of Rise of the Tomb Raider. *Game Studies* 20(3), 9.

Fiske, S. T. (2018). Stereotype Content: Warmth and Competence Endure. *Current Directions in Psychological Science* 27(2), 67–73. https://doi.org/10.1177/0963721417738825

Fiske, S. T., Cuddy, A. J. C., Glick, P., and Xu, J. (2002). A model of (often mixed) stereotype content: Competence and warmth respectively follow from perceived status and competition. *Journal of Personality and Social Psychology* 82, 878–902.

Fox, J., & Tang, W. Y. (2017). Sexism in video games and the gaming community. In *New Perspectives on the Social Aspects of Digital Gaming* (pp. 115–135). Routledge.

Fox, J., Bailenson, J. N., & Tricase, L. (2013). The embodiment of sexualized virtual selves: The Proteus effect and experiences of self-objectification via avatars. *Computers in Human Behavior* 29(3), 930–938. https://doi.org/10.1016/j.chb.2012.12.027

Fox, J., Ralston, R. A., Cooper, C. K., & Jones, K. A. (2015). Sexualized avatars lead to women's self-objectification and acceptance of rape myths. *Psychology of Women Quarterly* 39(3), 349–362. https://doi.org/10.1177/0361684314553578

Fredrickson, B. L., & Roberts, T. A. (1997). Objectification theory: Toward understanding women's lived experiences and mental health risks. *Psychology of Women Quarterly* 21(2), 173–206. https://doi.org/10.1111/j.1471-6402.1997.tb00108.x

Gestos, M., Smith-Merry, J., & Campbell, A. (2018). Representation of women in video games: A systematic review of literature in consideration of adult female wellbeing. *Cyberpsychology, Behavior, and Social Networking* 21(9), 535–541. https://doi.org/10.1089/cyber.2017.0376

Glennon, J., Johnston, D., Francisco, E. (May 14th, 2020). The Rest of Us: The Last of Us II Controversy Explained. *Inverse*, Retrieved 09/06/2025. https://www.inverse.com/gaming/last-of-us-2-trans-controversy-explained-abby-tlou

Glick P., Fiske S. T., Mladinic A., Saiz J. L., Abrams D., Masser B., . . . López W. L. (2000). Beyond prejudice as simple antipathy: Hostile and benevolent sexism across cultures. *Journal of Personality and Social Psychology* 79, 763–775. https://psycnet.apa.org/doi/10.1037/0022-3514.79.5.763

Glick, P., & Fiske, S. T. (1997). Hostile and benevolent sexism: Measuring ambivalent sexist attitudes toward women. *Psychology of Women Quarterly*, 21(1), 119–135. https://doi.org/10.1111/j.1471-6402.1997.tb00104.x

Goettner-Abendroth, H. (2018). Re-thinking 'matriarchy 'in modern matriarchal studies using two examples: The Khasi and the Mosuo. *Asian Journal of Women's Studies* 24(1), 3–27. doi: 10.1080/12259276.2017.1421293

Heflick, N. A., Goldenberg, J. L., Cooper, D. P., & Puvia, E. (2011). From women to objects: Appearance focus, target gender, and perceptions of warmth, morality and competence. *Journal of Experimental Social Psychology* 47(3), 572–581. https://doi.org/10.1016/j.jesp.2010.12.020

Hooi, R., & Cho, H. (2014). Avatar-driven self-disclosure: The virtual me is the actual me. *Computers in Human Behavior* 39, 20–28. https://doi.org/10.1016/j.schb.2014.06.019

HORIZON ZERO DAWN [Playstation 4] (2017). Crystal Dynamics.

Jagayat, A., & Choma, B. L. (2021). Cyber-aggression towards women: Measurement and psychological predictors in gaming communities. *Computers in Human Behavior* 120, 106753. https://doi.org/010.1016/j.chb.2021.106753

Kaye, L., Gresty, C., & Stubbs-Ennis, N. (2017). Exploring Stereotypical Perceptions of Female Players in Digital Gaming Contexts. *Cyberpsychology, Behavior, And Social Networking* 20(12), 740–745. https://doi.org/10.1089/cyber.2017.0294

Kelly, D., Nic Giolla Easpaig, B., & Castillo, P. (2023). 'You Game Like a Girl': Perceptions of Gender and Competence in Gaming. *Games and Culture* 18(1), 62–78. https://doi.org/10.1177/15554120221077730

Kim, C., Lee, S., & Kang, M. (2012). I became an attractive person in the virtual world: Users' identification with virtual communities and avatars. *Computers in Human Behavior* 28, 1663–1669. https://doi.org/10.1016/j.chb.2012.04.004

King, A. E., & Douai, A. (2014). From the "Damsel in Distress" to Girls' Games and Beyond: Gender and Children's Gaming. In *Gender Considerations and Influence in the Digital Media and Gaming Industry*, 1–17. IGI Global.

Kowert, R. (2020). Dark Participation in Games. *Frontiers in Psychology* 11. https://doi.org/10.3389/fpsyg.2020.598947

Lynch, T., Tompkins, J. E., Van Driel, I. I., & Fritz, N. (2016). Sexy, strong, and secondary: A content analysis of female characters in video games across 31 years. *Journal of Communication* 66(4), 564–584. https://doi.org/10.1111/jcom.12237

MacCallum-Stewart, E. (2014). "Take That, Bitches!" Refiguring Lara Croft in Feminist Game Narratives. *Game Studies*, 14(2). http://gamestudies.org/1402/articles/maccallumstewart

Maity, N. (2014). Damsels in distress: A textual analysis of gender roles in Disney princess films. *IOSR Journal of Humanities and Social Science* 19(10), 28–31.

McMenomy, E. R. (2011). *Game on girl: identity and representation in digital RPGs*. Washington State University.

Mikula, M. (2003). Gender and Videogames: the political valency of Lara Croft. *Continuum* 17(1), 79–87. https://doi.org/10.1080/1030431022000049038

Nightingale, E. (2021, June 1). Snowflake gamer dragged after whining about Aloy's 'masculine' appearance in Horizon Forbidden West. *Pink News*. https://www.thepinknews.com/2021/06/01/horizon-forbidden-west-aloy-masculine-sony-state-of-play/

Paaßen, B., Morgenroth, T., & Stratemeyer, M. (2017). What is a true gamer? The male gamer stereotype and the marginalization of women in video game culture. *Sex Roles* 76(7), 421–435. https://doi.org/10.1007/s11199-016-0678-y

Pfister, E. (2018). "In a world without gold, we might have been heroes!" Cultural Imaginations of Piracy in Video Games. In *FIAR: Forum for Inter-American Research*, 11(2).

Ramos, M., Barreto, M., Ellemers, N., Moya, M., & Ferreira, L. (2018). What hostile and benevolent sexism communicate about men's and women's warmth and competence. *Group Processes & Intergroup Relations* 21(1), 159–177. https://doi.org/10.1177/1368430216656921

RESIDENT EVIL 4 [GameCube] (2005). Capcom.

Salter, A., Blodgett, B. (2017). Come Get Some: Damsels in Distress and the Male Default Avatar in Video Games. In *Toxic Geek Masculinity in Media*. Palgrave Macmillan, Cham. https://doi.org/10.1007/978-3-319-66077-6_4

Smith, J. L., Sansone, C., & White, P. H. (2007). The stereotyped task engagement process: The role of interest and achievement motivation. *Journal of Educational Psychology*, 99(1), 99–114. https://doi.org/10.1037/0022-0663.99.1.99

Spencer, S., Logel, C., & Davies, P. (2016). Stereotype Threat. *Annual Review of Psychology* 67(1), 415–437. doi: 10.1146/annurev-psych-073115-103235

Stermer, S. P., & Burkley, M. (2012). SeX-Box: Exposure to Sexist Video Games Predicts Benevolent Sexism. *Psychology of Popular Media Culture*. Advance online publication. https://doi.org/10.1037/a002839

Summers, A., & Miller, M. K. (2014). From damsels in distress to sexy superheroes: How the portrayal of sexism in video game magazines has changed in the last twenty years. *Feminist Media Studies* 14(6), 1028–1040. https://doi.org/10.1080/14680777.2014.882371

THE LAST OF US PART II [Playstation 5] (2020). Naughty Dog.

TOMB RAIDER [Playstation 1] (1996). Core Design.

TOMB RAIDER [PlayStation 4] (2013). Crystal Dynamics.

Vandenbosch, L., Driesmans, K., Trekels, J., & Eggermont, S. (2017). Sexualized video game avatars and self-objectification in adolescents: The role of gender congruency and activation frequency. *Media Psychology* 20(2), 221–239. https://doi.org/10.1080/15213269.2016.1142380

Video Gaming Worldwide – Statistics and Facts (2023, August 31). *Statista*. Retrieved September 20, 2023, from https://www.statista.com/topics/1680/gaming/#topicOverview

Wells, G., Romhanyi, A., Reitman, J. G., Gardner, R., Squire, K., & Steinkuehler, C. (2023). Right-Wing Extremism in Mainstream Games: A Review of the Literature. *Games and Culture*, https://doi.org/10.1177/15554120231167214

Wojciszke, B. (2005). Morality and competence in person-and self-perception. *European Review of Social Psychology* 16(1), 155–188. https://doi.org/10.1080/104632805 00229619

Yao, M. Z., Mahood, C., & Linz, D. (2010). Sexual priming, gender stereotyping, and likelihood to sexually harass: Examining the cognitive effects of playing a sexually-explicit video game. *Sex Roles* 62, 77–88. https://doi.org/10.1007/s11199-009 -9695-4

Yoon, G., & Vargas, P. T. (2014). Know thy avatar: The unintended effect of virtual-self representation on behavior. *Psychological Science* 25(4), 1043–1045. https://do i.org10.1177/0956797613519271

# Through the Empty Bottles

## YouTube Comments as a Reaction Towards Depictions of Alcoholism in PSYCHONAUTS 2

*Tero Kerttula*

Many games have included using alcohol within the gameplay. However, very few games still discuss and depict the abuse of alcohol. Some media writings have discussed whether the depictions of excessive alcohol usage are glorifying alcoholism or not (e.g. Crecente 2012 & Hamilton 2019). This is a challenging question, as some games let the players have the characters consume alcohol within the game, while also either contributing to the storyline of the game or altering the game mechanics via the use of alcohol. Examples of such games are POSTAL 2 (2003), DEAD RISING 2 (2010), GRAND THEFT AUTO V (2013), KINGDOM COME: DELIVERANCE (2018) and most recently BALDUR'S GATE 3 (2023).

Only a few games, on the other hand, discuss and explore the concept of alcoholism within the narrative and through the characters. These games include such titles as PAPO & YO (2013), MAX PAYNE 3 (2012), LYDIA (2017) and AFTERPARTY (2019), which discuss the effects of alcoholism to the people and society around the alcoholics. This article is a study of a more recent game called PSYCHONAUTS 2 (Xbox Game Studios 2021). It is a video game released on multiple platforms in August 2021 as a direct sequel to the first game, which was released in 2005. The game is a platforming adventure which deals with some serious life issues throughout its stages, such as post-traumatic stress disorder (PTSD), depression and alcoholism.

Alcohol abuse seems to be a widely under-researched area in video game studies. The closest one to the topic of this study seems to be Jo Cranwell's and her associates' study about alcohol and tobacco content in video games (Cranwell et al., 2016). However, the theme has been researched and discussed more in cinema studies for a long period of time (see Herd 1986, Steudler 1987, Kanner 1990, Denzin 1991 & Cullum-Swan 1992).

Coming from the background of media and cultural studies, this article focuses on a certain chapter in PSYCHONAUTS 2 called "Bob's Bottles," which is directly about the mindset of an alcoholic and further tries to visualize what an alcohol-addicted mind might look like. The aim of this study is to look at (1) how the game portrays an alcoholic mind to the audience, and through that audience to see; and (2) how this portrayal is discussed and reacted to. The audience is looked at as a broad concept, where the audience is layered through YouTuber, the commenters, and the general audience.

This study investigates different layers of interpretation, which are created when the game is transferred into another medium, in this case YouTube Let's Plays, online streams and video essays. In these formats, the original game content becomes unplayable, and the audience is presented with new means of narration, which overlap the original story of the game. This study is also an exercise in using publicly available sensitive material in research without compromising the security and the personal information of the people commenting on
YouTube. A possible way of doing this is implemented within the study and tested with the research material. Because the story needs to be analyzed throughout, it needs to be noted that there are some story spoilers ahead for those who have not yet played the game.

## Theory and methodology

This study consists of two sections. The first part discusses the original narrative of the game in an attempt to see different discourses with which the game represents different aspects of alcoholism. This analysis is based on identified discourses around alcoholism (McFarlane & Tuffin 2010) and alcohol research in general. After that follows a brief look into ten different YouTube videos featuring the level Bob's Bottles. Two of the videos are video essays, which analyze the content of the section to the viewer. Two videos are non-narrated walkthrough videos. The rest of the videos are Let's Plays by three authors, which each divided the section into two different videos. The videos used in the study are as follows:

*Table 1: Videos used in the study*

| Author | Video Title | Genre |
|---|---|---|
| Mister Donlon | Psychonauts 2 and Addiction: Bob Zanotto | Video Essay |
| PurePari | Uncorking Bob's Bottles | Video Essay |
| MaterWelonz | Bob's Bottle – Psychonauts 2 Let's Play Part 22 & 23 | Let's Play |
| Mehdi Juventino Gaming HQ | Psychonauts 2 – 100%Walkthrough Part 19: Bob's Bottles | Walkthrough |

| Author | Video Title | Genre |
|---|---|---|
| Kakuchopurei | Psychonauts 2: Bob's Bottles Walkthrough \| SPOILERS | Walkthrough |
| Wanderbots | You're Fired! – Let's Play Psychonauts 2 – PC Gameplay Part 20 | Let's Play |
| Wanderbots | Bottom oft he Bottle – Let's Play Psychonauts 2 – PC Gameplay Part 19 | Let's Play |
| PlayFrame | Psychonauts 2- #20 – Vestige in a Bottle | Let's Play |
| PlayFrame | Psychonauts 2- #19 – Green Needle Gulch | Let's Play |

These creators were chosen for the analysis because their videos came out soon after the game's launch. While there are now a few other let's plays on YouTube, in the videos chosen for the study it is certain that the players are adventuring through the game for the first time. This section looks at how the narrators discuss with the game dialogue and how they discuss with their audience.

Lastly, the focus of the study is the comments left below the YouTube videos. As the subject matter of the study is sensitive through the personal mentions of alcohol abuse, some extra means to preserve the privacy of the commenters were created. The comments written in these videos were collected during six months, from September 2021 to March 2022. In that time, these videos gathered a total number of 842 comments. The analysis of the comments began by coding the comments with identifiers (Coffey & Atkinson 1996, 26–53). A total of 134 comments were identified as *commenting the theme and narrative of the game* and taken for further analysis. Other identifiers for the comments were *commenting the player-narrator*, *commenting the game mechanics*, *commenting other videos of the player-narrator* and *general commentary*. Most usually these comments featured inquiries from the YouTube persona of when a game the commenter wished to see would be played in the channel and therefore didn't contribute to the analysis much. These comments were deleted from the data after the identification process.

The remainder of the comments were taken to a second round of coding. Here, the comments were coded according to the visual elements in the gameplay and narrative that the commenters refer to. For example, mentions of bottles were coded accordingly. Some of these codes required further reading into the comment and the narrative. A prime example here is the mentions of vines and plants. In some cases, the commenters referred to the vines as just plants, even though these two elements serve completely different purpose in the narrative. Because of this, these conflicting mentions were coded according to the narrative rather than the explicit mention itself. After the general coding, the comments were analyzed further by their theme and discourse.

No personal information or recognizable pieces of information, such as nicknames, were collected. To further the anonymization of the comments, a certain method of hiding the identity of the commenters was created for this study. Instead of referring to the commenters with their screen aliases, they are referred to as [YC], in abbreviation for "YouTube commenter." The numbers after the YC tag in the comments quoted in this article have been randomized, so that the comments cannot be connected directly to any of the videos referred to in this study. The comments quoted in this study have also been altered with earlier mentions of alcoholism referred to as [alcoholism], [expression of alcoholism] and various other paraphrasing methods. Any mentions of family members in the shown data have been paraphrased as [family member]. This removes any implications of gender and relation between the commenter and the family member in question. The thought behind this follows Pierre Bourdieu's (1996) views of the family as a field (Goodsell & Seiter 2011, 320–323 & Atkinson 2014, 224–225) as regarding the study, the genders, connections, and relationships do not change the interpretation. Doing all this, the original content of the comment is still intact, but it cannot be found with search engines. This was proven by running a Google search through each of the comments after alteration. Longer comments are also referred to only partially, where the comment is only used as an example of the discourse discussed. The collected data will be stored on an external device after the study. This device will be stored in a locked compartment. The data will not get published and no digital copies of the data will be stored elsewhere, to protect the identity of the commenters.

One mention regarding the comments is that many videos regarding PSYCHONAUTS 2 had only a handful of comments underneath them. In many cases this was because the video was an upload of live-streamed content. Most of the commentary given to the player-narrators was instead during the live stream, which in addition gives this study a small caveat. In some Twitch.tv recordings, the chat is retained in the video, while in others, the chat has been removed. Furthermore, many of the comments collected were quite long and structured, the longest comments reaching up to 1,500 characters in length. In live-streaming environments, such as Twitch.tv, there is usually a character limit, and the pace of the live stream does not let the commenters share their insights long after the stream has been concluded.

There are several studies regarding YouTube comments on many fields. In one earlier study, a research group aimed to find if the comments affect the viewers of public service announcements considering marijuana use. Even though the research showed that the effect of the PSAs was dampened by these comments, the research group also wondered whether the effect was made by the comments or the YouTube environment in general (Walther, DeAndrea, Kim & Anthony 2010). Schultz, Dorner and Lehner (2013) created a classification system for YouTube comments, to see which comments would qualify as useful to use in for example research. In their data they found that a majority of the comments examined could be classified as "inferior," which the research group ponders to be one aspect of a certain bad image YouTube comments tend to have (Schultz, Dorner and Lehner, 2013). A certain study by Martin Roth (2022) examines the comments made on YouTube videos about ANIMAL CROSSING: NEW HORIZONS in context of the COVID-19 virus and the retaining of everydayness through the video content and the commentary on YouTube. Here Roth has lots of material to work with, and he refers to the comments as his own translations from Japanese to English. Roth also works his way through the comments by looking at certain keywords, from which the analysis continues (Roth 2022, 8–9).

The comments also contribute to the concept of audience regarding this study. Looking at Lets' Plays and other videos, there are several different audiences to be seen. The player-narrator is also audience to the game in question. The commenters are audience to the game and the player-narrator. In the bottom of this chain are us, viewing the game, the player-narrator, and the commenters. Of course, we could also be audience only to the game, or to the player-narrator, if the comment section is not read or if we were watching just a recording of the game or playing ourselves.

Regarding being audience also to the comments, it is assumable that the comments were not directed to the whole field of audience, but rather the player-narrator or select few other commenters. This is what for example Douglas Park (1982) refers to as the division between implied audience and actual audience (Park 1982, 249–250). The difference here between implied audience and intended audience is that in the videos, the script implies that there is an audience viewing the video. From one perspective, the intended audience could be just anyone, as of course the creators wish to have as broad an audience as possible to their videos (Strangelove 2010, 44). But within their narration they do imply that there are people behind their screens watching their antics. In the case of video game-based videos, this is also because they do not need to make the game they are playing desirable to play; instead, the player-narrators wish to make their own performance a desirable watch and therefore marketable (Kerttula 2022, 81–82). Also, even though only a handful of the viewers in a video participate in the discussion, many more share the video through their own social media channels, thus becoming participatory audience in their own way (Jenkins 2018, 21–22).

The different audiences here then involve the player-narrator, the commenters and people reading the comments as different types of audiences. This is also something that makes YouTube commentary unique and differentiates it from, for example, discussions on online forums. Even though people can be interacting with one another, there are several different levels of communication visible than just the discussing people themselves. Theorizing these multiple levels of audience here is crucial, as the Let's Play videos are very different from other kinds of YouTube content. Many YouTubers today communicate with their audience and encourage them to write down in the comment section. This kind of reflective narration is one of the features which make YouTube videos unique (Koskimaa 2019, 18–19).

## Bob's bottles and the notion of alcohol abuse

The narrative in the PSYCHONAUTS games works in two different narrative spaces. All the characters reside in the overworld, but their problems and issues are only confronted when literally diving into their minds. One of these characters whose mind the protagonist dives into is called Bob Zanotto, a short, bearded gardener who has isolated himself away from the other people and seemingly lives only with his plants and his memories. The segment tries to recreate an image of an alcoholic mind. The level features closed bottles, which Raz needs to open to dive deeper. These seemingly empty bottles contain Bob's memories, which are in each bottle and are related to his mother, his work and to his marriage. The visual aesthetic of the level gives not-so-subtle hints about the subject matter. The most notable ones are the bottles, which are used as platforms or other means of getting through the level. The bottles are also a part of the narrative.

The game makes the alcoholism of Bob's mother clear, as the story sees her constantly wandering into a greenhouse, where she spends peculiarly long periods of time. After a certain point in the stage, the game takes the protagonist into the said greenhouse, where he finds an abundance of empty, green bottles, giving a clear hint that Bob's mother was drinking in the greenhouse. Here the story explains that Bob's mother was hiding her bottles in different places around their home and the greenhouse, which is one of the oldest-known characteristics of alcoholism (see Simmel 1948). As the mother character is so heavily incorporated into the story, the narrative then makes a hint about the hereditary features of alcoholism. This feature of alcoholism has been studied extensively by Donald W. Goodwin (Goodwin 1979 & 1985). The study on this field is continuous even to this date, and even though there are some variables in the conclusions of the studies, there definitely seems to be a hereditary component in alcoholism (see Walters 2002 & Cox & Klinger 2022).

It is also worth pointing out how the game portrays a female character as an alcoholic. In popular culture, drinking women are more scarcely seen when compared to alcoholic men. According to earlier film studies, it is pointed out how female alcoholism is often portrayed through a relationship to a man (Kanner 1990, 184).

The first segment also tries to give subtle rhetoric explanations behind the alcohol abuse. One of these reasons, which carries over from mother to son, is loss and the grief related to it. The narrative gives hints about Bob's father falling in a battle, which is hinted as a cause for the mother to begin drinking. In the same vein, as the mother and later Bob's significant other passes away, Bob also tries to find relief and comfort in alcohol. Research seems to agree with this interpretation, as grasping the bottle when confronting loss is a well-studied reason behind drinking (Gold et al., 2000 & Eddinger et al., 2018).

The narrative through the segments of the level is carried by the need of finding certain flower seeds, which also contain parts of Bob's memories. Obtaining these seeds is made more difficult by an unnamed moth, which carries the seeds away in an attempt to hide them from Raz. The identity of the moth is revealed to be Bob in disguise, which in part discusses how parts of Bob don't want these difficult emotions and events in his life to be raised up again. This then concerns a well-known feature of alcoholism, that being denying the drinking and telling lies about it, with feelings of guilt and shame related to the problem involved (Black 1979; Smith 1998 & de Beaurepaire 2014). To back this interpretation up, shame in particular is also evidently seen in the segment featuring Bob's mother, as her facial expressions can be seen as sad and guilty (Figure 2). Bob also only learns about his mother's drinking after her death, when visiting the said greenhouse. Thus, the mother had kept her drinking hidden from her offspring. The denial later involves Bob personally, as he denies his problem in the narrative in a dialogue with Raz.

*Figure 2: Expression on the face of Bob's mother (right) as she leaves to the greenhouse*

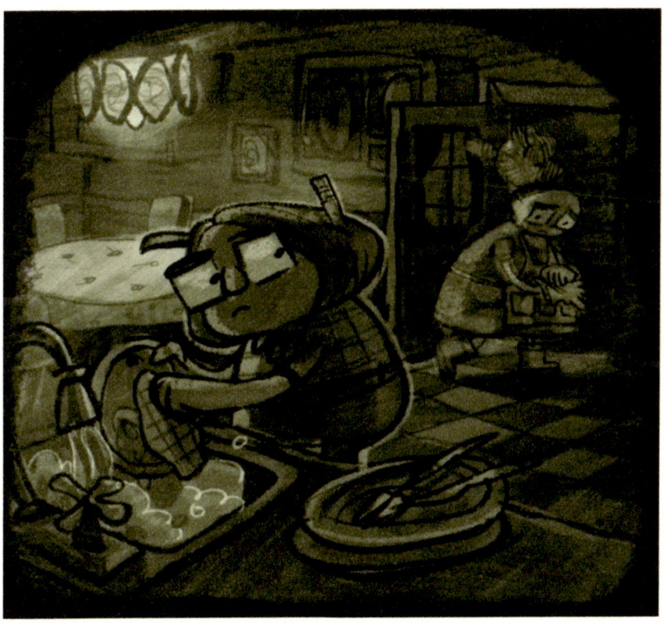

This can lead to something called a circle of suffering, which was explored in Brian A. Smith's phenomenological study about the suffering alcoholism can cause to an individual (Smith 1998, 216). Denying the problem, while still having it, can lead to a self-destructive behavior where one starts to lean towards the addiction whenever problems occur in life, while at the same time pushing people away and slowly starting seclusion from one's surroundings.

Bob is portrayed as a kind of recluse, all alone on a small island inside his mind. Inside there are other characters from the game, or rather representations of them, as the characters only visually resemble their counterparts in the game world. The character's dialogue consists of how Bob perceives other people seeing him. For example, in one certain scene in the level, Bob gets fired from the Psychonauts because of his drinking by a character called Truman Zanotto. On the islands, we can find Truman only repeating the line, "You're fired!" with an angry tone, whereas in the bottled memory, Truman tears up while doing this and tries to give Bob a number to an assumed help line or such, which Bob consequently refuses. This is an interesting narrative feature, as research seems to suggest that letting an alcoholic employee go is not necessarily the right way to handle the situation; offering treatment should be the first action. Nevertheless, many alcoholics do end up losing their jobs (Singh & Sindolya 2022 251–252 & Trice & Beyer 1984, 393–395).

One certain visual detail in the level is the use of pink. At the beginning of the level, the visuals are dominated by green, blue, and brown tones. However, as Raz proceeds through the level, the tones start to vary, and especially at the last part, the sky and the clouds turn pink. This, in my opinion, refers to the "pink cloud syndrome." Pink clouds are usually connected to recovering from alcoholism, where the person recovering from alcohol addiction begins to feel like being inside a pink cloud (e.g., Richards & Bascue 1978, 15; Spiegel & Fewell 2001, 131–132).

As a visual choice, this is interesting, because we see the pink clouds at a part which concerns Bob's marriage. They are also somewhat present in the first section, but not as dominant. These pink clouds might then refer to the character recovering from his initial alcoholism via his marriage. This angle is supported by the fact that the player character is literally inside Bob's memory of his wedding, thus supporting the interpretation that Bob remembers this time through the rose-tinted glasses of these pink clouds. As research shows (Richards & Bascue, ibid.), slipping away from this pink phase to drinking again is usual, which in Bob's case is evident, as pink cannot be seen throughout the remainder of the level after the wedding.

## Let's Plays and the comments

A Let's Play (LP) is a written text or an online video where a player narrates the experience of playing a game from the viewpoint of oneself (Kerttula 2019, 237–238,

Svelch & Svelch 2022, 1098). This then leads to this player-narrator creating a story about playing the game, overlapping the original story of the game (Kerttula 2022, 72). An important thing here to notice is that the player-narrators are also audience to the original game. Especially when doing a blind Let's Play, the player-narrators show constant emotional responses to the game, be that laughs, sighs or something else. In the LPs of PSYCHONAUTS 2, we can hear many ways of expressing emotions towards the story of the game and even some explicit mentions of the reactions the story raises:

> [PlayFrame]: "I guess I could use the salts. I think he might've have a like...Bob, Bob's mother might have had some alcoholism going on, it sure seems that way. But a lot of these figments are telling a bit more of the story too and suggesting that he might've uh, he might have inherited that."

The video essays portray a different tone. As the narration is not immediate and is certainly written beforehand, they also serve a different purpose in the analysis of the game. However, the video essays are not without their emotional parts:

> [Mister Donlon]: "This moment will pull your heartstrings later, when you realize that agent Zanotto despite his rant earlier, is actually a soft-spoken, sensitive person, who last lost many of the people closest to him throughout his life."

The essays also have numerous rhetorical questions, in which the narrator ponders alternate versions of the scenario presented in the game:

> [Mister Donlon]: "This brings up a divisive subject for alcoholism. Was it right to fire Bob for being unable to control his problem, or could there've been another answer?"

Mister Donlon also educates his audience about alcoholism with several bits of information concerning alcohol use disorder (AUD). These issues are not explained thoroughly, even though there are for example mentions of Wernicke-Korsakoff syndrome, which is a serious condition of thiamine deficiency, and the twelve-step program of Alcoholics Anonymous (AA).

> [Mister Donlon]: "The idea for his mind to be a mostly ocean to traverse, is a nod to what psychologist refer to as Wernicke-Korsakoff Syndrome, or wet brain" & "The reasons he has AUD are also areas he needs to focus on for his treatment. There's similar logic that goes into Alcoholics Anonymous and the twelve step program, actually."

Sari Piittinen (2018) makes a notice about the moral evaluations of the player-narrators, in which she brings up the possibility of pre-writing and emotional exaggeration for the entertainment of the audience (Piittinen 2018). The latter can be found from the video essay by PurePari, as he mostly sticks to narrating the plot of the game and analyzing the story. This essay also features a line in which the narrator expresses the emotion he has towards the scene in question, which even though is clearly pre-written, is also expressed in a very reactionary way, differentiating the line from the rest of the narration:

> [PurePari] "I'm not crying, you are crying!"

When it comes to the comment section, initially the coding was started at the gameplay level. For example, if the commenter mentioned or analyzed the stream of flowers or the moth, these comments were coded accordingly. This was to see if the comments correlate with the narration of the video. At this core the most mentioned feature was the bottles (n=31). Other core-level mentions in the comments were the moth (n=12), the plants (n=10), the vine (n=7), the seeds (n=8), the flowers (n=2) and the pink clouds (n=2). The plants and the vine are different entities in the narrative, the vine being an active participant in helping the player, while the plants are used only as platforms or such. In some comments, these two were mixed, so the coding was done analyzing the comment as a whole. In shorter comments, these and the other core-level mentions were often paired with short insights into what meanings might have been put in said visual narrative element. For example, in a video where the narrator ponders the moth and what it represents multiple times, there are numerous answers in the comments section to the question through the commenter's own interpretation of the moth:

> [YC84] "The moth represents alcoholism."

Only three commenters expressed that they hadn't understood that the level was about alcoholism. These comments were also paired with expressions of laughter and humor. Few commenters also displayed their dismay and disgust towards alcohol use:

> [YC79] "Lol didn't realize he was alcoholic until this video. These things really go over my head"

> [YC107] "Get drunk or play video games? The answer for me is the latter. I don't understand why people like getting drunk or alchohol in general."

From here, the analysis continued with the recognized references to the features of alcoholism. One distinct recognized feature of alcoholism was the hereditary nature of alcoholism. As PSYCHONAUTS 2 depicts Bob's mother as a problem drinker, the game explores the hereditary aspects of alcoholism through the storyline. Regarding this, there were no explicit mentions in the comments about female alcoholism. The hereditary aspects of alcoholism were recognized by several commenters (n=11) in a general manner:

> [YC43] "...of course [alcoholism] is a hereditary thing."

The hereditary alcoholism was also mentioned by many commenters, who wrote about their relatives with drinking problems. In some comments it was specifically mentioned how the commenter specifically avoids alcohol because of their alcoholic relatives.

> [YC86] "[representation of alcoholic character] is significant because alcoholism can be genetic. [YC expressing caution towards alcohol] because I have a long family history of alcoholism..."

Another thing rising from the comments is the mentions of Bob being secluded, introverted and how he is "pushing people away" (n=9). These comments are mostly paired with a mention of the bottles or the moth, but in all cases, they seem to address the game environment as a metaphor for seclusion. In addition, a few commenters pondered the possibility of the islands being a metaphor for how Bob drove people away. This was perceived by some commenters, who recognized the depression in the depiction of the character.

> [YC42] "[Reacting to a depiction of Bob's depression]...This was a very accurate way to show the mind of a depressed alcoholic. Bottles everywhere, I mean everywhere."

> [YC13] "It's because he pushes everything away in his attempt to protect himself from the pain of severed bonds of attachment."

Some aspects were not commented on that often. Refusing the offered help (n=5) and denial of the problem (n=2) especially gathered fewer comments. However, only looking at the amounts here is not crucial. The most interesting thing is how commenters connect these observations to their own lives. For example, looking at the aspect of hiding the bottles, which was also mentioned only a handful of times (n=6), the content of the comments is all about the lived experience of the commenter:

> [YC73] "My [family member] was in a similar situation. [Family member] would always hide alcohol in...random cabinets."

This brings up a very important discourse repeating in the data, which is the discourse of family. This is because some commenters explicitly mentioned for example their parents being alcoholic, while in some comments, the concept of family is less clear, as the commenters only refer to the persons in question as family. In some comments (n=18), the commenters reflect their own experiences with alcoholic relatives, while others (n=29) discussed the hereditary features of alcohol abuse from different angles. As the section in the game deals with alcoholic lineage, this result is something to address further. These comments are often paired with the discourse of grief (Ord 2009, 197–201), as the commenters bring across the struggle and sadness of living with an alcoholic relative.

> [YC79] "... seeing the way [alcoholism] tore [family members] lives apart..."

> [YC112] "...being sober for a long time because [family member] finally recognized the pain [expression of alcoholism] was causing himself and others."

A number of commenters (n=4) also wrote about their own struggles with addiction. Two of these comments were very long, structured commentaries on how living as an addict feels, whereas two comments were shorter, but not without content:

> [YC42] "[Expression of addiction recovery] this level was especially compelling for me as I could somewhat relate to what Bob was going through."

This kind of depiction of an alcoholic mind seems to have had an impact, then. The commenters who have encountered alcoholism from family or from their own use seem to have a shared experience of identification with the setting and the characters from the game. This leads to a key finding from the comments, which is that regardless of the type of video, empathy is expressed toward Bob's character and the other characters found in the level as well (n=43). These comments can be long, structured ones or just short expressions of the writers' feelings.

> [YC44] "[Expression of empathy]... Bob's in serious pain and for a long time it seems..."

> [YC73] "[Expressing of empathy]...That Bob would rather hide his memories, and thus his needing to deal with them, behind his alcoholism."

Empathy, as Kristie S. Fleckenstein (2007) argues, always involves an element of rationality. This is because the person expressing empathy recognizes the suffering of the other (Fleckenstein 2007, 702). In the context of PSYCHONAUTS 2, it is then arguable that the commenters expressing empathy do have an idea or an experience of what alcohol abuse is like and what it causes. This is especially visible in the comments where the discourse of family and self are present, in this sense because the experience has been personal.

Some of these empathetic reactions seem to stem from Bob's character being presented as a lonely, suffering person, leading to many of the commenters explicitly mentioning Bob's pain and the character's need to hide that pain behind alcohol, at the same time making matters worse. In other cases, the commenters tried to find justification behind some of the actions seen in the level, such as Truman letting Bob go from his work.

One thing to be noted is that the commenters in these videos could be subscribers to the channel they are commenting on. This means that the people commenting have watched several other videos by the same author and in some comments, it seems that they experience a certain bond with the narrator. This is an important note, as feeling familiar with the narrator could lead to a feeling of a safe environment to comment in. In this case, the familiarity also makes it easier to write comments about more personal issues. How video games convey empathy in different manners has been discussed a lot in research (see Ho and Ng 2022, 1187), but in this case, the expressions of empathy are not coming from the player, but rather from someone watching someone else play and react to the actions.

Therefore, the conversations between the commenters and the narrator were also identified and coded. Comments which were coded as *conversation_video* refer to the commenters discussing with the narrator, or making certain observations from the narration, which are then directed towards the narrator. In turn, comments which were aimed towards other commenters in the same section were coded as *conversation_comm*. These are hard to identify, as many of the more analytical comments could act as a continued analysis from the one present in the video, but the commenters do not address the narrator directly. This is also in many cases hard to identify from the tone of the comment.

> [YC74] "Hey [mention of narrator], um, I don't know that Bob's mom was merely an alcoholic...Based on how you were talking about it, I thought maybe I should say something because you maybe want to take a second look, just in case there was a misunderstanding there."

This is also where the concept of audience comes in and especially the theories around implied audience and actual audience. First and foremost, most of the viewers do not comment under the video. For example, MarzGurl's video featured in this study gathered over 80,000 views by the time of gathering the data, but only 49 comments. As many of the comments were directed to the narrator and the other commenters, the publicity of the written comment becomes a more difficult notion. As the actual audience to the comments, we are subject to many tough stories of people's lives, but not as the implied audience. The comments are made to reflect something that both the game and the video made the commenter ponder upon. What is also noticeable from this is that there are no comments that could be considered as negative or hateful towards the narrator or the game characters.

When it comes to the commenters reacting to other comments, there is no simple way of pointing out which comment made someone react in some way. However, when the comment section of a video gets looked as a whole, the tone of the commentary and the different reactions between the commentators and the narrator become more evident. Comments about personal issues result in more personal comments in the section. The tone and length of the comments also seem to differ between the different types of videos. Generally, the comments made on the video essays were longer and more analytic, whereas the comments made on the Let's Plays are shorter and more like instant reactions. As a result, comments made on video essays discuss more the analysis itself, while other comments are made more towards the player-narrator and game. As an important mention, since the videos aside from the video essays are divided into two parts, so are the comments. This in turn leads to the commenters reacting to the events in each video and only rarely reflecting the events from the previous video.

## Conclusion

It seems that this section of the game wanted to tell a story about an alcoholic individual while giving insight into the mind of a person suffering from a substance abuse. The features of alcoholism in the game seem to be recognized somewhat well by both the YouTubers and their audience, then, even though some of the more obvious features stand out from the data. The most important things here are how the recognitions often come from experience about substance abuse from family or from one's own life. This leads to a notable portion of the comments having a discourse of empathy. The empathetic reactions are varied, but they seem to share the same kind of view from a fictional person's perspective, thus making the commenters feel the way the writers probably wanted to. From a game writing point of view, looking through comments of some YouTube videos could turn out to be a good way to see what kind of writing works for the audience. This also applies to watching the videos themselves.

The most notable result is the way commenters discuss their own lives in reflection to the events in the game and the player-narrator. They also discuss these events with one another. It seems that a familiar narrator and an identity hidden behind an alias creates a safe environment in which to express emotions and ideas that come from one's life. This is supported by the number of empathetic comments as well.

This study was also used to test how online comments should be anonymized when used as research data. In the context of this study, the method applied here seems to be effective and does not compromise the private information or security of individual commenters. This is because the comments were treated only as a textual data, no private information was collected, and all connections to the material was made vague. The downside of this is that the integrity of the data can suffer as a result, and comments made under a single video file are more difficult to compare to each other. This method of anonymization should be tested further on different data to see if there are any other downsides or compromises to it.

From the viewpoint of the concept of the audience rises an important note: as the Let's Plays broaden the audience of the game to those who have not played the game, the message the game is conveying also gets a larger audience, but with new layers of interpretation. The commenters who have not played the game interpret the game narrative through the player narrative. Also, people who do not comment, but watch and read the comment sections, get many ulterior views into the original message of the game.

## References

Atkinson W. (2014) A sketch of 'family' as a field: From realized category to space of struggle. *Acta Sociologica* 57(3), 223–235. https://doi.org/10.1177/0001699313511470

Benzies L. (2013) GRAND THEFT AUTO V (Playstation 4 version) [Video game] Rockstar Games.

Black C. (1979) "Children of Alcoholics." *Alcohol Health and Research World* 4(1).

Bourdieau P. (1996) On the Family as a Realized Category. *Theory, Culture and Society* 13(3).

Caballero V. (2012) PAPO & YO (PC Version) [Video game] Minority Media Inc.

Coffey A. J. and Atkison P. A. (1996) *Making Sense of Qualitative Data: Complementary Research Strategies*. London: Sage.

Cox W. M. and Klinger E. (2022) Genetics of Alcoholism. In *Why People Drink; How People Change*, edited by W. Miles Cox & Eric Klinger, 39–50. Cham: Springer.

Cranwell J., Whittamore K., Britton J. and Leonardi-Bee J. (2016) Alcohol and Tobacco Content in UK Video Games and Their Association With Alcohol and Tobacco Use Among Young People. *Cyberpsychology, Behavior and Social Networking* 19(7). https://doi.org/10.1089/cyber.2016.0093

Crecente B. (2012) "Max Payne 3 Is a Character Study Shaped by Addiction and Violence." *Polygon*, Polygon, 30 Apr. 2012, https://www.polygon.com/gaming/2012/4/30/2988059/Max-payne-3-is-a-character-study-shaped-by-addiction-and-vi olence.

Cullum-Swan B. (1992) The Alcoholic in Films: Self or Other? Symbolic Interaction 15(2). https://doi.org/10.1525/si.1992.15.2.241

de Beaurepaire R. (2014) "The use of very high-doses of baclofen for the treatment of alcohol-dependence: a case series." *Frontiers in Psychiatry* 10. https://doi.org/10.3 389/fpsyt.2014.00143

Denzin, N. K. (1991) *Hollywood Shot by Shot. Alcoholism in American Cinema*. London: Routledge.

Eddinger J. R., Humiston T. M., Sutton M. L., Jobe-Shields L. and Williams J. L. (2019) Alcohol Use and Drinking Motives Among Suddenly Bereaved College Students, Journal of Dual Diagnosis, 15:1, 16–24, https://doi.org/10.1080/15504263.2018.1531185

Fleckenstein, K. (2007) "Once Again With Feeling: Empathy in Deliberate Discource". *JAC* 27(3/4). https://www.jstor.org/stable/20866807

Gold J., Neururer J. and Miller M. (2000) Disenfranchised Grief among First-Semester Male University Students: Implications for Systemic and Individual Intervention. *Journal of the First-Year Experience & Students in Transition* 1(21).

Goodsell T. L. and Seiter L. (2011) Scrapbooking: Family Capital and the Construction of Family Discource. *Journal of Contemporary Ethnography* 40(3). DOI: 10.1177/0891241611399437

Goodwin D. W. (1979) Alcoholism and Heredity. A Review and Hypothesis. *Arch Gen Psychiatry* 36(1). DOI: 10.1001/archpsyc.1979.01780010063006

Goodwin D. W. (1985) Alcoholism and Genetics. The Sins of the Fathers. *Arch Gen Psychiatry* 42(2). DOI: 10.1001/archpsyc.1985.01790250065008

Hamilton J. (2019) "Are Video Games Glorifying Alcoholism?" *Informa* (blog). *Game Developer*. August 20, 2019. https://www.gamedeveloper.com/business/are-vid eo-games-glorifying-alcoholism-

Herd D. (1986) Ideology, melodrama and the changing roles of alcohol problems in American films. *Contemporary Drug Problems* 213(1986).

Ho J. C. F. and Ng R. (2022) Perspective-Taking of Non-Player Characters in Prosocial Virtual Reality Games: Effects on Closeness, Empathy, and Game-Immersion. *Behaviour and Information Technology* 41(6). DOI: 10.1080/0144929X.2020.1864018

Jenkins H. (2018) Fandom, Negotiation and Participatory Culture. In Booth P (ed.) *A Companion to Media Fandom and Fan Studies*. John Wiley and Sons Inc. New Jersey, USA.

Kanner M. (1990) That's Why the Lady Is a Drunk: Women, Alcoholism and Popular Culture. In Raymond D (ed.). *Sexual Politics and Popular Culture*. Bowling Green State University Popular Press. Ohio, USA.

Kerttula T. (2019) "What an Eccentric Performance": Storytelling in Online Let's Plays. *Games and Culture*, 14(3), 236–255. https://doi.org/10.1177/155541201667872 4

Kerttula T. (2022) (Broad)casting the Game: The Spectacle of Real in Representing and Narrating Video Game Play. University of Jyväskylä. https://jyx.jyu.fi/handl e/123456789/79213

Koskimaa R. (2019) Game of Thrones -pelin Let's Play -videot ja populaarikulttuurin vastaanotto esityksenä. Lähikuva, 32(3), 7–25. https://doi.org/10.23994/lk.87955

Krankel S. (2019) AFTERPARTY (PC Version) [Video game] Night School Studio LLC.

Kuprejanov S. (2012) MAX PAYNE 3 (Xbox 360 version) [Video game]. Rockstar Games.

LYDIA (PC version) [Video game] (2017). Alko Oy.

McFarlane A. and Tuffin K. (2010) Constructing the Drinker in Talk about Alcoholics. *New Zealand Journal of Psychology* 39 (3): 46–55.

Ord R. L. (2009) "IT'S LIKE A TATTOO": Rethinking Dominant Discources on Grief. *Canadian Social Work Review 26(2)*. https://www.jstor.org/stable/41669912

Park D. P. (1982) The Meanings of "Audience". College English 44(3).

Piittinen S. (2018) Morality in Let's Play narrations: Moral evaluations of Gothic monsters in gameplay videos of Fallout 3. *New Media & Society*, 20(12), 4671–4688. https://doi.org/10.1177/1461444818779754

Richards T. M. and Bascue L. O. (1978) Emotional Stages is Wives of Alcoholics During the Descent and Recovery Process of Alcoholism. *Journal of Drug and Alcohol Education* 23(2). https://www.jstor.org/stable/45091339

Riedel M. J. (2003) POSTAL 2 (PC Version) [Video game] Whiptail Interactive.

Roth M. (2022) Reclaiming Everydayness and Japanese Cultural Routines in *Animal Crossing: New Horizons. Journal of Intercultural Studies.* https://doi.org/10.1080/072 56868.2022.2134318

Schafer T. and McClendon Z. (2021) PSYCHONAUTS 2 (Xbox Series X version) [Video game]. Xbox Game Studios.

Schultz P., Dorner V. and Lehner F. (2013) Leave a comment! An In-depth Analysis of User Comments on YouTube. *Wirtschaftsinformatik Proceedings* 2013. http://aisel. aisnet.org/wi2013

Singh D. P. and Sindoliya M. (2022) Alcoholism: A Health and Social Evil. In Shanwal, Vinod K. & Chhikara B. S. (ed.) *Alcoholism. Causes, Symptoms, Effects and Treatment.* CRC Press. Oxon.

Simmel E. (1948) Alcoholism and Addiction. *The Psychoanalytic Quarterly* 17(1).

Smith B. A. (1998) The problem drinker's lived experience of suffering: an exploration using hermeneutic phenomenology. *Journal of Advanced* Nursing 27(1). https://do i.org/10.1046/j.1365-2648.1998.00524.x

Spiegel B. R. and Fewell C. H. (2001) 12-Step Programs as a Treatment Modality. In Ashenberg Straussner, Shulamith L. (ed.) *Clinical Work with Substance-Abusing Clients.* Guildford Press. New York & London.

Steudler F. (1987) Representations of Drinking and Alcoholism in French Cinema. International Sociology 2(1). https://doi.org/10.1177/026858098700200104

Strangelove M. (2010) Watching YouTube: Extraordinary Videos by Ordinary People. University of Toronto Press. Toronto, Canada.

Svelch J. and Svelch J. (2022) "Definitive playthrough": Behind-the-scenes narratives in let's plays and streaming content by video game voice actors. *New media and society* 24(5). https://doi.org/10.1177/1461444820971778

Trice H. M. and Beyer J. M. (1984) Work-Related Outcomes of the Constructive-Confrontation Strategy in a Job-Based Alcoholism Program. *Journal of Studies on Alcohol* 45(5). https://doi.org/10.15288/jsa.1984.45.393

Vávra D. (2018) KINGDOM COME: DELIVERANCE (Playstation 4 version) [Video game]. Deep Silver.

Vince S. (2023) BALDUR'S GATE 3 (PC version) [Video game] Larian Studios.

Wallace R. (2010) DEAD RISING 2 (Xbox 360 version) [Video game] Capcom.

Walters G. D. (2002) The Heritability of Alcohol Abuse and Dependence: A Meta-Analysis of Behavior Genetic Research. *The American Journal of Drug and Alcohol Abuse* 28(3). https://doi.org/10.1081/ADA-120006742

Walther J. B., DeAndrea D., Kim J. and Anthony J. C. (2010) The Influence of Online Comments on Perceptions of Antimarijuana Public Service Announcements on YouTube. *Human Communication Research* 36(4). https://doi.org/10.1111/j.1468-2958.2010.01384.x

# The Sanity Metre
## Madness as a Manageable Resource

*Stefan Heinrich Simond*

Resource management is a concept that is applied wherever limited resources must be allocated with careful deliberation. These limited resources can be the working hours of team members when assigning tasks or an annual budget that needs to be allocated to maximise profit. Resource management operates on the premise that achieving any particular goal requires efficiency (Townsend). Commonly, notions of resource management would be found in fields such as economics, financial administration, human resources, but also in political theory[1] and in environmental considerations.[2] Here, the term is applied to constructions of madness in video games, specifically in the case of the sanity metre—a status indicator of a character's mental constitution.

The sanity metre deserves particular attention as a construction of madness since it is exclusive to interactive systems. Linear media such as films or literature do not have any necessity for a sanity metre, whereas video games tend to integrate madness functionally into the games' rule system. This chapter argues that the sanity metre (1) renders madness operationalisable for a game's code, (2) has its historical roots in psychiatric discourse and its cultural roots in cosmic horror, and (3) that it presents players with contradictory affordances that require deliberate resource management.

Accordingly, the first section will offer a discussion on the *quantification* of mental health in the history of psychiatry, followed by an exploration of the roots of the sanity metre in cosmic horror[3]. The key focus is then a comparative analysis of three video games that more or less explicitly feature a sanity metre: AMNESIA: THE DARK DESCENT (Frictional Games, 2010), HELLBLADE: SENUA'S SACRIFICE (Ninja Theory,

1 See for example John Rawls' (1999, 58 ff.) integration of Pareto optimality into the social contract.

2 See for example Lawler et al. (2010).

3 The term 'horror' will not be explored further in this article. For a concise exploration see Therrien (2009).

2017), and TOKYO DARK: REMEMBRANCE (Cherrymochi, 2019). In all three titles, the sanity metre is described regarding its narrative, aesthetic, and ludic properties.[4]

Before getting to the central argument, I wish to briefly illustrate why and how the term 'madness' is used in this article as it can seem counterintuitive at best and derogatory at worst. Aside from a "serious mental illness," The Longman Dictionary defines 'madness' as "very stupid behaviour that could be dangerous or have a very bad effect" (LONGMAN DICTIONARY OF CONTEMPORARY ENGLISH). The term is often used colloquially—as in 'Are you mad?'—and it carries a derogatory connotation that cannot be ignored. However, there are three advantages to using the term 'madness' here: (1) There is an ongoing process of reclaiming the term, i.e., to imbue it with an empowering connotation in the context of personally affected people. This can be observed, for example, in the annual mad pride parade (Schaarschmidt). (2) It ties into a broader sociological and philosophical discourse. In his notable engagement *MADNESS AND CIVILIZATION*, Michel Foucault described a history of madness and expanded the meaning of madness from an individual ascription to the structural configuration of society as such. More recently, a strand of so-called 'mad studies' has emerged that presents a critical engagement with the psychiatric ascription of 'mental illness' and considers itself a form of 'survivor research'[5] (Beresford; Beresford and Russo). (3) Most importantly, madness opens up the field of enquiry. By using the term here, I wish to indicate that I am not referring to specific psychiatric diagnoses. The medical angle is one possible option to think about madness, but it is not the only one. Especially when engaging with constructions of madness in the media, it can be limiting to apply medical terminology. Since this article is not concerned with the application of actual diagnoses but rather with the historical and cultural significance of the sanity metre from a perspective of video game studies, the term 'madness' provides a sufficiently broad and abstract framework in which a range of different perspectives can be included.

## The quantification of mental health

At the core of any sanity metre is a *quantification* of mental health. This idea of assigning a quantitative measurement to a person's mental constitution is not particularly

4 This article builds upon some of the crucial findings presented in my PhD dissertation, titled PIXELATED MADNESS. THE CONSTRUCTION OF MENTAL ILLNESSES AND PSYCHIATRIC INSTITUTIONS IN VIDEO GAMES. Some key terms in this article are written in italics, such as *quantification, somatic externalisation*, etc. This indicates that they are types of madness that are directly tied to the sanity metre. For the full typology see Simond (in press).

5 An especially notable application of mad studies to HELLBLADE: SENUA'S SACRIFICE has been presented by Netchitailova (2019).

new. The earliest precursors in this domain can be traced back to Hippocrates' humoral theory, developed around 400 BC in his essay ON THE SACRED DISEASE, which was then further developed in Galen's ON THE NATURAL FACULTIES in the 2nd century (Merenda; Wampold 71; Franke 59; Farreras 3–4). Hippocrates and Galen describe four bodily fluids: blood, phlegm, yellow bile, and black bile. Depending on how these four fluids are distributed, a person might have a particular character or suffer from a particular affliction. Kalachanis aptly states: "Health absolutely requires the correct humor proportions. Consequently, humor excesses and/or shortages trigger the pathophysiology of disease." (2) This required balance must be maintained or restored; in other words, a healthy person manages their bodily fluids in a homeostatic equilibrium[6].

Another early example of quantification in a field that is adjacent to psychiatry is the concept of physiognomy as developed by Johann Caspar Lavater. Similar to humoral pathology, the quantity of somatic aspects is crucial. In the case of physiognomy, the measured quantity entails structural features of the face and skull. Lavater claimed that one could ascertain the character of a person by measuring and interpreting the outline of their head: "A forehead full of irregular protuberances is characteristic of a choleric temperament" (Lavater/Porta, 1817).

In contemporary psychiatry, humoral theory and physiognomy have no credible bearing. This does not mean though that the logic of *quantification* has vanished. Rather, it is applied in a different form. Contemporary *quantifications* may, for example, build upon the 'diathesis stress model,' which is commonly applied in the domain of allergology and psychology (Franke, 2012, p. 159).[7] The key idea is that people inevitably encounter 'stressors' throughout their life. Such stressors can be biomedical pathogens such as viruses or bacteria, but also distressing parts of daily life such as job insecurity, the loss of a loved one, or loneliness. In order not to fall ill, a person then requires 'resources' to process the stress. Such resources can be a smoothly operating immune system, but also supportive social relationships, passions and routines, or professional therapeutic guidance. The more resources one manages to acquire, the more resilient one is in the face of impending stressors.

*Quantifications* of mental health are also applied in specific therapeutic contexts, for example in the application of a perceived stress scale (PSS) (Lee). The PSS is used for patients of emotionally unstable personality disorder (EUPD), also known as borderline personality disorder (ICD-F60.3), and other afflictions that entail emotional dysregulation. The PSS quantifies the perceived stress level in numerical values. One

6 A "homeostatic equilibrium is the tendency of an organism or a cell to regulate the internal conditions." (Biology Online, 2019) A healthy organism thus manages to maintain stable even though the environment might change or adversely affect it.

7 A variation of this concept is the acronym 'HEDE,' which stands for 'health-ease' and 'dis-ease' as two opposing poles (Franke, 2012).

may then identify their base stress level, different thresholds that warrant the applications of skills, such as grounding or breathing exercises, and peak stress levels that mark the danger of losing control.[8] Notable here is the close proximity between the application of PSS in actual psychiatric care and the construction of the sanity metre in video games as detailed below.

## The roots of the sanity metre in cosmic horror

A formative occurrence of a sanity metre in the context of games is CALL OF CTHULHU by Chaosium (1981). The board game includes a rule system whereby characters lose sanity points when confronted with the supernatural. It is arguably no coincidence that a board game adaptation of the short story THE CALL OF CTHULHU (1928) by H.P. Lovecraft popularised the sanity metre. Indeed, there are identifiable thematic ties between the sanity metre and key ideas of cosmic horror.

THE CALL OF CTHULHU follows an unnamed protagonist who goes through a series of documents he inherited. He learns about a strange cult worshipping an ancient being called 'Cthulhu.' As part of their worship, the cult enacts peculiar rituals that are documented throughout history. An expedition by a group of sailors leads to the hidden city of R'lyeh in which Cthulhu awakes from its slumber, kills most of the crew, and leaves the few survivors bereft of their cognitive faculties. The story concludes with the author detailing how the mere knowledge of Cthulhu's existence suffices to drive people insane. The implication is that the entire world is at the hands of an incomprehensible deity that may destroy it at any given point.

The thematic tie to the sanity metre can be identified in the confrontation with the incomprehensible. THE CALL OF CTHULHU details several occurrences in which ancient secrets challenge or destroy reason. For example, the sailors that venture into the city of R'lyeh are assaulted by such incomprehensible sights that the few survivors hardly dare to recount the events. As Cthulhu eventually appears, the diegetic author narrates: "Everyone listened, and everyone was listening still when It lumbered slobberingly into sight and gropingly squeezed Its gelatinous green immensity through the black doorway into the tainted outside air of that poison city of madness" (Lovecraft, 1928). THE CALL OF CTHULHU is thus a story about the attempt to fathom the unfathomable. The cosmic forces of ancient deities are simply beyond the capabilities of human comprehension. Consequently, the fragility of reason is emphasised as even hardened explorers are driven mad. The sanity metre fulfils a similar function on a structural level. It constructs reason and madness as two opposing

8 The application of the PSS differs somewhat between countries though there are studies that intermittently evaluate the consistency and validity of PSS in the respective region. For one such study in Germany see Klein et al. (2016).

types, facilitates a conflict between the two, and characterises reason as fragile since encounters with madness lead to its depletion. Maintaining some degree of sanity then becomes a winning condition. As Garrad (2021, p. 26) puts it: "To be Sane, in the game's terms, is to be victorious."

Since its implementation in the 1981 board game, the sanity metre has been adapted in a variety of titles.[9] These include other licensed tie-ins in the Cthulhu Mythos, such as CALL OF CTHULHU: DARK CORNERS OF THE EARTH (Headfirst Productions, 2005) and CALL OF CTHULHU (Cyanide, 2018). However, the sanity metre has since received much wider recognition. Both ETERNAL DARKNESS: SANITY'S REQUIEM (Silicon Knights, 2002) and AMNESIA: THE DARK DESCENT have significantly contributed to the popularisation of the sanity metre—the latter is analysed in detail below. Other titles that implement a sanity metre are DON'T STARVE (Klei Entertainment, 2013), DARKEST DUNGEON (Red Hook Studios 2016), CRUSADER KINGS III (Paradox Development Studio, 2020), and INDIGO PROPHECY (titled FAHRENHEIT in Europe, Quantic Dream, 2005). A particularly prominent example is THE SIMS 4 (Maxis, 2014), which includes an expansive mood system as well as a character trait that was originally called 'insane,' but has been renamed 'erratic' in 2018 due to public criticism (Jackson 2018a, 2018b). Considering the prominence of the sanity metre in video games, it is important to ponder what its key narrative, aesthetic, and ludic properties are.

## The sanity metre in video games

The key function of a sanity metre is to render the abstract notion of madness operationalisable for the rule system (Vozaru, 2022, p. 65). A video games' rule system is constituted in the code, which operates according to specific parameters. Much in the sense of Niklas Luhmann's system theory, such a rule system is operationally closed, i.e. the rule system can only process information that adheres to its own logic (Luhman, 2000, pp. 25–35). In other words, for madness to be computed on the structural level of the game, it needs to be coded in the language of rules. While the sanity metre is not necessarily the only way to accomplish this, it is an established method.[10] On a most general level, this form of *quantification* is rather consistent with the way in which mental health is quantified within psychiatric discourse, especially in the case of PSS. Importantly though, the numerical values and calculations may well be concealed in the black box of the game. The code processes the values without them being immediately obvious to the player. Instead, the sanity

9 For a brief overview see Milesi (2022, 194 ff.).

10 After all, video games have been measuring health in general since their inception. For a deeper engagement with the *quantification* of health see Rogers (2020).

metre comes with an interface that communicates the sanity value to players by employing audiovisual representations. These can include icons, colours, audio cues, haptic feedback, etc.

Such audiovisual representations alert the player that the sanity value is tracked in one way or another. Consequently, players have to adapt their engagement with the game and its rule system to accommodate the sanity value. This is where the aspect of resource management literally comes into play. How exactly the sanity metre facilitates madness as a manageable resource and how this in turn affects player engagement is best explored in case analyses.[11]

### *Amnesia: The Dark Descent*

AMNESIA: THE DARK DESCENT (subsequently abbreviated as AMNESIA) is a survival horror game by the Swedish studio Frictional Games. It was initially released on 8 September 2010 for PC and later ported to consoles. AMNESIA quickly gained traction in the community of video game streaming and sold over 1.4 million copies by 2012 (Reilly). Due to its critical and commercial success, a series of sequels followed, such as AMNESIA: A MACHINE FOR PIGS (The Chinese Room, 2013), AMNESIA: REBIRTH (Frictional Games, 2020), and AMNESIA: THE BUNKER (Frictional Games, 2023). The title not only employs a rather conventional sanity metre but also popularised it beyond the licensed CALL OF CTHULHU games.

AMNESIA follows the journey of Daniel, an aspiring archaeologist, who wakes up in the Prussian castle of Brennenburg in 1839. He finds a note by his former self, stating that he erased his own memory and that he must find and eliminate the resident Baron Alexander. Throughout his exploration of the castle, Daniel is haunted by a horrid shadow from which he can only flee or hide. He also suffers from nyctophobia, i.e. pathological fear of the dark. Daniel gradually comes to understand that the aforementioned shadow began haunting him after he had discovered a mysterious orb at an excavation site in Algeria. Daniel is then contacted by Baron Alexander who promises to dispel the shadow in exchange for Daniel's servitude. Unbeknownst to Daniel however, Baron Alexander is trapped in an alternate dimension and requires the orb to return. He deceives Daniel and demands increasingly atrocious acts of him including torturing and killing villagers to infuse the orb with sufficient energy for Alexander to make his escape. As Daniel discovers Alexander's deception and realises the extent of his acts, he is overwhelmed by guilt and uses a potion to erase his own memory. Ultimately, Daniel confronts Alexander in the castle's Inner Sanc-

---

11 The following chapters contain narrative summaries include story spoilers for the three respective games AMNESIA: THE DARK DESCENT, HELLBLADE: SENUA'S SACRIFICE, and TOKYO DARK: REMEMBRANCE.

tum, and depending on player choices either Daniel dies, Alexander dies, or both are consumed by the shadow.

Within this narrative framework, the sanity metre plays a crucial role. It comes with the central components of resource management alongside Daniel's physical health. The shadow that haunts Daniel is encountered repeatedly throughout the game, and as soon as Daniel looks at it, the sanity value starts rapidly depleting. The implementation of the sanity metre can thus be interpreted as a ludic manifestation of the Lovecraftian notion that encounters with the incomprehensible are an existential threat to the faculties of reason (Garrad, 2021, pp. 21–23). This introduces a crucial complication on the ludic level for which *AMNESIA* is widely known. On the one hand, players must know the location of the shadow to effectively escape its clutches. On the other hand, players must avert the avatar's gaze as much as possible to avoid expending sanity. In other words, AMNESIA presents two contradictory actions by virtue of rendering sanity a resource to be managed and can thus evoke a sense of pressure and dread.

A similar effect is attained with Daniel's nyctophobia. To replenish sanity, Daniel must make progress with his exploration. However, he must also manage his lantern oil, lest he be engulfed by darkness. Venturing off the beaten path poses the risk of running out of oil, but also comes with the hope of finding more. Thereby, AMNESIA creates a sense of urgency (Schwager, 2012, p. 5). As Thon (2021, p. 204) points out: "the game mechanics force the player to constantly weigh the goal of not being seen by monsters against the goal of not losing sanity by lingering in the darkness."

*Figure 1: The four stages of sanity in AMNESIA: THE DARK DESCENT*

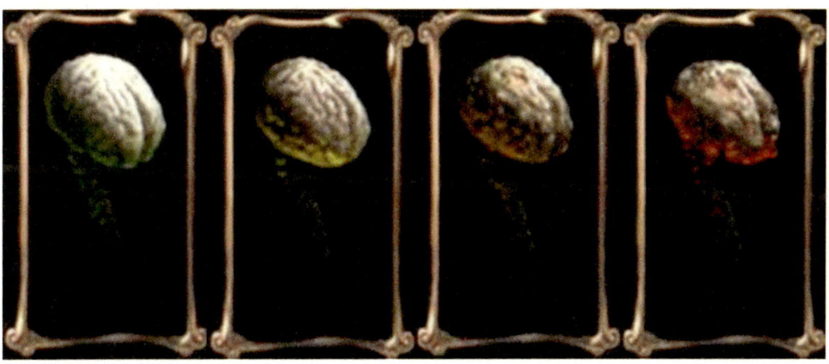

(Grip, 2014)

These considerations of resource management are additionally complicated by the fact that AMNESIA obscures the exact sanity value from players. The sanity metre is nested in the inventory screen. Instead of a concrete number or scale, players see one of four icons as depicted in figure 1. They combine two means of *externalisation*: (1) The icons are colour-coded from green, for entirely sane, to red, for an impending mental breakdown. The means of expressing the degree of madness in the form of colour may be referred to as a *visual spatial externalisation* of madness. (2) The icons also depict a central nervous system which is increasingly affected by lesions. In this way, AMNESIA presents a *somatic externalisation* that equates the loss of sanity with organic dysfunctionalities, much in the sense of how mental afflictions have historically been considered 'brain diseases' (Schneider, 1987, p. 7; Franke, 2012, pp. 70–71).

Another indicator of Daniel losing sanity is not found in the inventory but affects the character's perception. For instance, when Daniel's sanity drops below a certain threshold, his vision becomes blurry, and he begins to experience hallucinations. One such hallucination involves cockroaches crawling across the screen. They can be clearly discerned from diegetic reality since their location is relative to the camera movements, i.e. if players look around, the cockroaches will move along as if they sat on a virtual camera lens (Thon, 2021, pp. 204–205). According to Tom Reiss, these effects can instil a fear of fear itself, potentially plunging Daniel into a downward spiral of insanity. These hallucinations are *visual spatial externalisations* of madness and they clearly relate a *subjective* experience of losing one's mind. This is to say that they aim to immerse players in the experience of madness.

## *Hellblade: Senua's Sacrifice*

HELLBLADE: SENUA'S SACRIFICE (subsequently abbreviated as HELLBLADE) is a psychological action-adventure game developed by British studio *Ninja* Theory. After having worked with major publishers on accomplished titles such as HEAVENLY SWORD (2007), ENSLAVED: ODYSSEY TO THE WEST (2010), and DMC: DEVIL MAY CRY (2013), Ninja Theory advanced on their own terms by financing the development of HELLBLADE entirely without a publisher. HELLBLADE'S commercial success is largely attributed to its dedication to *radically subjectify*[12] the experience of psychosis, including voice-hearing and de-realisation. The developers consulted with mental health advisors as well as personally affected people. In 2018, Microsoft acquired Ninja Theory who have since released a sequel, titled SENUA'S SAGA: HELLBLADE II (2024). HELLBLADE takes a rather indirect and metaphorical approach to the sanity metre with a metadiegetic twist.

12 *Subjectification* in this context means that players experience the game from the perspective of a character coded as 'mad.' A *subjectification* is considered *radical* when this perspective is the only available perspective, i.e. if there is no way of discerning between what is diegetically real and what is not (Simond, in press).

HELLBLADE is set in the late 8th century and tells the story of Senua, a Pict warrior who travels to Helheim to revive the soul of her beloved, Dillion. Throughout her journey, Senua confronts mythological creatures that are tied to her experiences of trauma. She grapples with the imposing voice of her father, Zynbel, who had her mother, Galena, burned at the stake. A host of other voices speak to Senua and the player respectively, guiding them, but also diminishing their efforts or deceiving them. Senua explores the wilderness, identifies patterns in her environment, and fights against an onslaught of shadow warriors that are apparent reflections of the Northmen that pillaged her home and killed her beloved. Ultimately, Senua seems to fall in combat against Hela, the goddess of death. She survives, however, by acknowledging the need to let go of her grief. Senua drops Dillion's decapitated head into an abyss and invites the player to come along since there is yet another story to tell.

Strictly speaking, HELLBLADE does not feature a sanity metre because it abstains entirely from an interface with numbers and icons. This is consistent with HELLBLADE'S approach to *radically subjectify* madness, i.e. to exclusively focus on Senua's personal experience. Any conventional interface such as an inventory, damage numbers, or even a health bar would literally stand between Senua and the player as well as reduce the complex subjectification presented to a series of numbers. There is, however, a mechanic in HELLBLADE that approximates the function of a sanity metre and can be interpreted as a metaphorical abstraction thereof: the 'dark rot.'

*Figure 2: At the beginning of HELLBLADE, Senua is infected with 'dark rot' which gradually grows up her arm each time she is defeated in combat*

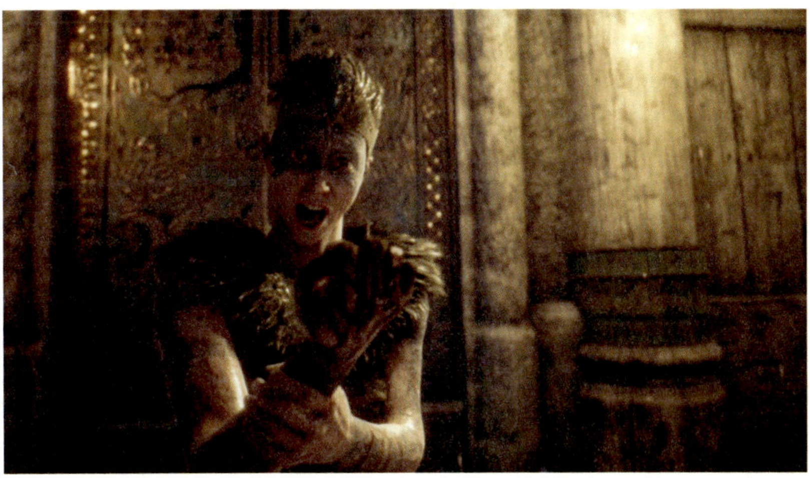

Screenshot by Author

After the introductory sequence, Senua stands before a locked gate that blocks the path toward Helheim. Behind her, several shadow Northmen appear and a combat tutorial ensues. While players learn the ropes of combat, Senua ultimately collapses and is consumed by dark rot.[13] A diegetic narrator voice announces that Senua being consumed by the rot is a vision of the future. Senua stands over her own body and sees how the rot begins to creep up her arm while she scratches it and screams in fear (fig. 2). A textual insert reads[14]:

The dark rot will grow each time you fail
If the rot reaches Senua's head, her quest is over
and all progress will be lost

This threat is actually empty. HELLBLADE does not feature a permadeath mechanic and no save data is ever erased, regardless how many times players fail. Before going into detail on the functional level though, it is first warranted to consider how the dark rot in HELLBLADE fulfils the function of a sanity metre and how it is tied to the history of madness. It has been mentioned already that a sanity metre operates with quantifications on the level of code, but that it must not necessarily express itself in the user interface in numbers or scales. While it can only be speculated how exactly the dark rot is tracked in HELLBLADE, it appears likely that there is an invisible number that increases each time Senua is defeated in combat. Corresponding to each number is the advancing rot. As such, the dark rot operates as a manageable resource that needs to be kept at a minimum by investing the warranted degree of focus in each combat encounter.

Aesthetically, the dark rot is tied to the historical association between madness and infectious skin diseases. As Michel Foucault details in MADNESS AND CIVILIZATION, many facilities that later housed 'the insane' were initially built to confine the medieval outbreak of leprosy (in Gutting, 2012, p. 52). The bacterial infection became a serious threat that spread rapidly throughout the population due to limited facilities of public hygiene. Its most iconic symptom consists of skin lesions that may cause severe tissue damage as well as deformations, especially of the extremities (Rosen, 2015, p. 25). Once the epidemic died down and the leprosories stood empty, they were repurposed as general hospitals and confinement facilities in which, amongst others, 'the insane' were interned. Foucault illustrates how the literal stigma of leprosy carried over to the 'insane':

---

13 As may have become apparent already, battles that cannot be won are a recurring theme in HELLBLADE. Regarding the final combat encounter in the game, Berge (2021, p. 42) states that "this moment reinforces the central message of Senua's psychological struggle, as the player must—like her—accept the loss they have avoided for so long."

14 This is also the only textual insert in the entire game aside from the credits.

What doubtless remained longer than leprosy, and would persist when the lazar houses had been empty for years, were the values and images attached to the figure of the leper as well as the meaning of his exclusion, the social importance of that insistent and fearful figure which was not driven off without first being inscribed within a sacred circle.

HELLBLADE picks up on this historical association by *somatically externalising* Senua's experience of madness as dark rot. This entails several components that can each be considered a part of the interpretation: (1) Senua experiences herself as vulnerable and under constant threat of being consumed. This is expressed in the dark rot as a persistent reminder of her fear. (2) Senua's father, Zynbel, considered her to be cursed by 'the darkness.' In several flashbacks throughout the game, Zynbel warns Senua against giving into the darkness lest she be consumed by it. In this sense, the dark rot is a manifestation of the supernatural understanding that Senua's father imposed upon her. (3) Senua is further traumatised by the invasion of the Northmen. In her absence, they pillaged her home and burned the remaining inhabitants. The metaphor of bodies being consumed by fire is repeated several times throughout the game. For example, as Senua makes her way to face Surt, the god of fire, the path is lined with piles of smouldering corpses. The dark rot is visually related to burned skin, which demarcates her colonised subjectivity (Shelve, 2019). (4) Lastly, the dark rot is a reminder of the grief Senua experiences. Each time she falls at the hands of the perpetrators that sacrificed her beloved, her literal scar becomes more apparent. This interpretation is also supported by the ending of the game. When Senua eventually learns to let go and drops Dillion's head, the dark rot fades. Though Senua is not 'cured,' she comes to terms with her loss. Senua also learns to reject her father's understanding of the darkness and confronts her fears. In both of these instances, Senua is liberated from an oppression that haunted her.

As stated above, the threat of erasing save data is actually empty. Arguably, such a permadeath mechanic would seem out of place in a story-based game such as HELLBLADE. This fake permadeath mechanic can be considered deceptive game design, which Gualeni and Van de Mosselaer define as "the deliberate attempt to misguide players' inferences about the designer's intentions." (1) Assuming that players have not read an article that spoils the deception—such as this one—this threat would likely change their approach to combat encounters. The dark rot is then linked to a precious non-diegetic resource: the players' time investment into the game. This can be considered a *ludic actional externalisation* of madness because Senua's experience of madness affects how players engage with the game and its systems (Berge, 2021, p. 41; Meakin and Vaughan, 2021). On the matter of the sanity metre, Christopher and Leuszler (2022, p. 14) point out that "the sensation of collapse between the horror of the game narrative and the reality of the gamer will be all the more terrifying."[15]

15 Bernard Perron (2005) makes similar observations on the manner in which fear is conveyed.

On a metadiegetic level, the permadeath mechanic could even be considered especially effective precisely because it does not exist. Players may experience a sense of tension while playing that is not substantiated by an actual threat. The fear of losing progress is a fabrication, which equates to the experience of Senua being afraid of things that others might not consider to be real. This dynamic can be described as a *transdiegetic disruption* because it transgresses the boundaries of diegesis to involve the player as a player—and raises the question of who is playing with whom.

## *Tokyo Dark: Remembrance*

Tokyo Dark: Remembrance is an extended version of Tokyo Dark (jp. 東京ダーク, Cherrymochi, 2017), a psychological horror point-and-click adventure game with visual novel elements and a branching narrative that is largely contingent on player choices. The game was crowdfunded on Kickstarter and has been ported to Nintendo Switch and PlayStation 4 since its initial release on PC in 2017. Subsequently, the title will be abbreviated as Tokyo Dark, though the version played for analysis was Tokyo Dark: Remembrance on Nintendo Switch. The title engages deeply with the theme of madness and constructs not just one but two sanity metres, both of which warrant cautious resource management.

In Tokyo Dark, Detective Itō Ayami investigates the disappearance of her partner, Kazuki Tanaka. Tracking his whereabouts to the sewers in Shinjuku, Itō finds her partner brutally murdered by a woman named Reina. Itō shoots Reina and suffers a mental breakdown from which she awakens several weeks later. Increasingly obsessed with finding out more about Reina, Itō explores the underbelly of Tokyo and the surrounding areas. Ultimately, she finds that Reina's parents partook in a mass suicide ritual in Aokigahara (also known as 'Sea of Trees') to infuse Reina with ominous powers. Reina later commits suicide, yet cannot traverse to the beyond. Killing Itō's partner and several other people was Reina's attempt at obtaining a mask to open 'The Door' that would grant her passage. Throughout the investigation, Itō not only struggles with bullying and social exclusion at the police department, but also loses hold of her sanity. Depending on the choices made, Tokyo Dark leads to one of eleven endings. Here are just a few examples: Itō may help Reina pass on; she may overdose on medication; she may join her partner in the beyond, or the entire adventure is revealed as a silly plot devised by her cat, Lady Fluffington, who is actually a god.

The sanity metre in Tokyo Dark is part of the so-called 'SPIN' system, which is an acronym for Itō's four character attributes that can be checked in the inventory: **S**anity, **P**rofessionalism, **I**nvestigation, and **N**eurosis (fig. 3). All four attributes are consistently tracked and displayed as numerical scales from -100 to +100. Professionalism tracks how seriously Itō takes her role as a police detective. It rises when Itō asks deliberate questions based on evidence and falls when she acts brashly, emotionally, or violently. If professionalism is at a low value, players can choose more options to break the law and if the value is high, other characters are more respectful towards Itō. Investigation tracks how thoroughly Itō explores her surroundings. The higher the value is, the more clues will be revealed as more options for interaction become available.

*Figure 3: After having a mental breakdown, the hospital nurse explains the workings of the SPIN system to Itō and the player respectively in* TOKYO DARK: REMEMBRANCE

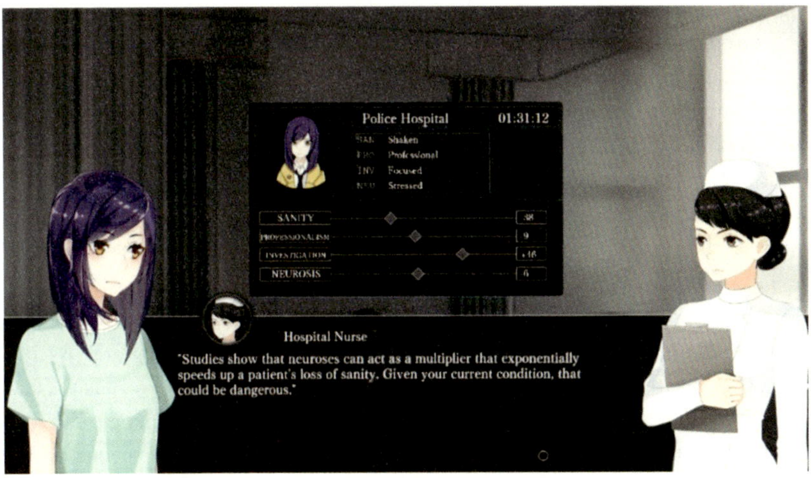


Screenshot by Author

Sanity operates as a conventional sanity metre, not unlike in the analysis of AMNESIA. Itō is inevitably confronted with emotional distress, disturbing occurrences, and ultimately the occult. For example, when Itō explores an abandoned section of the sewers and the lights suddenly go out, her sanity drops by -5. If Itō's sanity value reaches -100 by the time she enters Aokigahara, the narrative concludes that Itō is a patient in a mental institution and that the entire investigation has been a delusion. There are means to replenish sanity, though, for example by engaging in kind interactions, making time to relax, or taking medication. Replenishing sanity may come with other adverse effects, however. For example, taking medication increases sanity by +10 but, presumably as an implication of side effects, decreases the investigation value by -10. Players are thus discouraged from simply taking as much medication as they desire to 'adjust' the sanity value.[16]

From everything described so far, the sanity metre in TOKYO DARK is a conventional form of resource management. Consistent with the observations made for the case of AMNESIA, the sanity metre in TOKYO DARK requires players to carefully consider the choices they make. In keeping with the Lovecraftian notion of madness, sanity is constructed as being adversely affected by encounters with the incomprehensible. In contrast to AMNESIA as well as HELLBLADE, though, the player's aim in TOKYO DARK must not necessarily be to keep the sanity value as high as possible. At least if players wish to unlock all of the endings, they must manage sanity as a resource also by deliberately expending it to the degree that certain narrative branches require. The aim then becomes to drive Itō moderately or severely insane and watch the chaos unfold that comes with some of the available endings. Since TOKYO DARK follows a cyclical structure and partly refers to previous playthroughs, such approaches can be considered an affordance of the game design. Therefore, Garrad's (2021, p. 26) observation on CALL OF CTHULHU—"To be Sane, in the game's terms, is to be victorious."—does not apply to TOKYO DARK. Instead, one may choose to indulge in any degree of insanity to explore the story to its fullest.

An interesting complication is introduced with the fourth attribute, though, that has not yet been addressed: neurosis. The term is adapted from Freudian psychoanalysis and associated with the concept that people may repress certain desires that then manifest in psychopathological syndromes. The most apt type of neurosis that could be applied to TOKYO DARK concerns obsessive-compulsive behaviour, which includes "the irresistible entry of unwanted ideas, thoughts, or feelings into consciousness or [...] the need to repeatedly perform ritualistic actions that the sufferer perceives as unnecessary or unwarranted" (Britannica, n.d.).

In TOKYO DARK, neurosis measures the degree to which the player engages in meaningless repetition. The neurosis value increases by repeatedly speaking to the same character, even though they have nothing new to say, or by pacing back and forth between locations without any progress in the investigation. Crucially, the neurosis value operates as a modifier for the sanity value in inverse proportionality. This means that the higher the neurosis value grows, the lower the sanity value drops and the harder it becomes to increase it. The neurosis metre is of much significance here since it incorporates performative player actions into the game's construction of madness as *ludic actional externalisation*. Especially in point-and-click adventures with some degree of puzzle solving, it is customary player behaviour, when stuck

16 The way in which psychopharmacological medication is presented in TOKYO DARK would warrant much critical reflection. This point is left aside here though to focus specifically on the sanity metre.

with a puzzle, to talk to all the characters again or randomly interact with seemingly insignificant objects. TOKYO DARK incorporates these generally non-narrative interactions into its system of resource management, thereby encouraging players to think more cautiously about how to progress with the investigation. This leads to a complication that takes players as players into account.

## Conclusion

The key focus of this article was to analyse how the sanity metre renders madness into a manageable resource. From a genealogical viewpoint, it is notable that mental health has been quantified in psychiatric discourse and its historical predecessors in various ways. In video games, this *quantification* serves the primary purpose of rendering an abstract notion of madness operationalisable for the rule system. Since the rules embedded in the game code can only process what is compatible with its language, such *quantifications* are the functional basis of resource management.

Analyses of games have shown that sanity metres employ forms of *externalisation* to present the sanity value with audiovisual means. TOKYO DARK is most simplistic in this domain by displaying a numerical value alongside a slider. Whenever the protagonist's sanity value is modified, a pop-up appears that details the exact number of points lost or gained. TOKYO DARK therefore makes the underlying calculations transparent. The other analysed titles conceal such numerical values. AMNESIA employs a colour-coded icon that depicts a central nervous system. As the sanity value depletes, the central nervous system is increasingly affected by lesions. This form of directly associating madness with the physicality of the brain can be referred to as a *somatic externalisation*, i.e. it 'projects' the abstract notion of madness onto the body and its organs. HELLBLADE follows a similar trajectory but instead of focusing on the brain, it *somatically externalises* madness in the form of 'dark rot.' The dark rot can be interpreted as a combination of Senua's trauma, the mythology of darkness, and the historical association between madness and leprosy.

By rendering the sanity value a functional part of the games' rule system and by communicating it to players via an aesthetically externalised interface, the sanity value becomes a crucial component of the way in which the game is played. This effect is referred to here as a *ludic actional externalisation* since it presents specific affordances that players must take into account. In the course of the three analyses presented above, it has been found that the sanity metre primarily complicates player interaction with contradictory affordances that warrant resource management.

In AMNESIA, the primary directive is to advance through the castle swiftly to conserve and replenish sanity. Since the lantern oil is limited, though, players are strongly encouraged to explore their surroundings lest they be engulfed by darkness. Even more apparent is the contradiction between having to locate the ominous shadow that haunts the protagonist while having to avoid looking at the shadow since every glance rapidly depletes the protagonist's sanity.

TOKYO DARK encourages a more playful engagement with the sanity value. In order to experience the games' many endings, players have to expend sanity and drive the protagonist to a mental breakdown. Further, TOKYO DARK complicates player interaction by introducing a second value—the neurosis value—that renders otherwise common player behaviour, such as repeatedly speaking to characters or investigating random objects, a crucial factor in the resource management. Accordingly, TOKYO DARK instructs players to take the diegetic investigation seriously and consider their next move with caution.

HELLBLADE takes a similar approach and combines it with what may be called a *transdiegetic disruption*, i.e. its dark rot mechanic transcends the diegetic boundaries and addresses the player as player. This is accomplished by the game threatening players that their save data will be erased should the sanity metre reach its maximum value. If players care about not losing progress, they would engage in each combat encounter with caution. Curiously, the threat is fake, which adds another layer to the interpretation. Since players might be constantly worried about losing progress without any objective threat, their heightened state of anxiety corresponds to the diegetic sense of dread Senua experiences. Through deceptive game design, Ninja Theory provides a rather unconventional form of *radically subjectifying* the experience of madness.

These observations provide an initial vantage point on the significance of the sanity metre in video games, especially on its historical and cultural roots as well as its narrative, aesthetic, and ludic functions. By considering madness as a manageable resource, the sanity metre renders an abstract and elusive phenomenon a crucial part of reasonable considerations that in turn present specific and often contradictory affordances to players. The analysed titles here are but a few examples, though; and for further study it would be exceedingly helpful to build a database of games that feature a sanity metre to enable more systematic analyses. Especially considering that the sanity metre is one of the few aspects in which video games crucially differentiate their constructions of madness from linear media, further enquiries seem warranted.

## References

Beresford, P. (2020). "Mad", Mad Studies and Advancing Inclusive Resistance. *Disability & Society*, vol. 35, no. 8, 2020, 1337–42.

Beresford, P. and Russo, J. (Eds.) (2022). *The Routledge International Handbook of Mad Studies*. Routledge, Taylor & Francis Group.

Berge, P. S. (2021). Rotten and Possessed: Control and Hellblade: Senua's Sacrifice as Models of Outmersive Game Design. *Proceedings of the 32st ACM Conference on Hypertext and Social Media*, 35–44.

Biology Online (2019). *Homeostatic Equilibrium*. https://www.biologyonline.com/dictionary/homeostatic-equilibrium

Britannica. *Neurosis*. https://www.britannica.com/science/neurosis

Christopher, D. and Leuszler, A. (2022). Horror Video Games and the 'Active-Passive' Debate. *Games and Culture,* Special Issue: Reflecting and Evaluating Game Studies.

Farreras, I. (2013). *History of Mental Illness*. In Robert Biswas-Diener and Ed Diener (Eds.), DEF Publishers, https://nobaproject.com/modules/history-of-mental-illness

Franke, A. (2012). *Modelle von Gesundheit und Krankheit*. Huber.

Galen (2006). *On the Natural Faculties*. Edited by Arthur John Brock, Reprinted, Harvard University Press.

Garrad, J. (2021). Gamifying Fictions of Defeat: Adaptations of Lovecraft in Games Media. In Franz J. Potter et al. (Eds.), *The Popular and the Weird: H.P. Lovecraft and Twenty-First-Century Adaptation*, 21–9. Cardiff University Press.

Grip, T. (2014). *Game Design Deep Dive: Amnesia's 'Sanity Meter.'* https://www.gamasutra.com/view/feature/223931/game_design_deep_dive_amnesias_.php

Gualeni, S. and Van de Mosselaer, N. (2021). Ludic Unreliability and Deceptive Game Design. *Journal of the Philosophy of Games*, 3(1), 1–22.

Gutting, G. (2012). Foucault and the History of Madness. *The Cambridge Companion to Foucault: Second Edition*, 49–73. Cambridge University Press.

Hippocrates. (400AD). *On the Sacred Disease*. The Internet Classics Archive, translated by Francis Adams. http://classics.mit.edu/Hippocrates/sacred.html

Jackson, G. (2018a). The Sims Developers Quietly Rename the Game's 'Insane' Trait. *Kotaku*. https://kotaku.com/the-sims-developers-quietly-rename-the-game-s-insane-1825469692

Jackson, G. (2018b). The Sims' Insane Trait Sucks. *Kotaku*. https://kotaku.com/the-sims-insane-trait-sucks-1823590379

Kalachanis, K. (2015). The Hippocratic View on Humors and Human Temperament. *European Journal of Social Behaviour*, 2(2), 1–5.

Klein, E. M., et al. (2016). The German Version of the Perceived Stress Scale – Psychometric Characteristics in a Representative German Community Sample. *BMC Psychiatry*, 16(1), 159.

Lavater, J. C. and della Porta, G. (1817). *The Pocket Lavater, or, the Science of Physiognomy*. Van Winkle & Wiley. https://www.gutenberg.org/cache/epub/57030/pg57030-images.html

Lawler, J. J., et al. (2010). Resource Management in a Changing and Uncertain Climate. *Frontiers in Ecology and the Environment*, 8(1), 35–43.

Lee, E.-H. (2012). Review of the Psychometric Evidence of the Perceived Stress Scale. *Asian Nursing Research*, 6(4), 121–27.

Longman Dictionary of Contemporary English. *Madness*. https://www.ldoceonline.com/dictionary/madness

Lovecraft, H. P. (1928). *The Call of Cthulhu*. hplovecraft.com/writings/texts/fiction/cc.aspx

Luhmann, N. (2000). *The Reality of the Mass Media*. Polity Press.

Meakin, E. and Vaughan, B. (2021). "Understanding" Narrative; Applying Poetics to Hellblade: Senua's Sacrifice. *Game Studies*, 21(2). https://gamestudies.org/2102/articles/meakin_vaughan_cullen

Merenda, P. F. (1987). Toward a Four-Factor Theory of Temperament And/or Personality. *Journal of Personality Assessment*, 51(3), 367–74.

Milesi, L. (2022). Mind Games: Affective Ludo (Bio) Technologies of Fear. *Parallax*, 28(2), 195–212.

Netchitailova, E. (2019). The Mystery of Madness through Art and Mad Studies. *Disability & Society*, 34(9–10), 1509–15.

Perron, B. (2005). Coming to Play at Frightening Yourself: Welcome to the World of Horror Video Games. *Aesthetics of Play*, 14–15.

Rawls, J. (1999). *A Theory of Justice*. Revised Edition, Belknap Press of Harvard University Press.

Reilly, J. (2012). Amnesia Sales Pass One Million. *Game Informer.* https://www.gameinformer.com/b/news/archive/2012/09/10/amnesia-sales-pass-one-million.aspx

Reiss, T. (2015) "The Only Thing We Have to Fear Is Fear Itself": Horror as a Semiotic Medium in Amnesia: The Dark Descent. *Münchner Semiotik*, 2015.

Rogers, B. (2020). "Dude, How Much Health Do You Have Left?": On Masculinity and the Rationalization of Health in Video Games. In Arno Görgen and Stefan H. Simond (Eds.), *Krankheit in Digitalen Spielen. Interdisziplinäre Perspektiven*, 325–44. transcript.

Rosen, G. (2015). *A History of Public Health*. Revised expanded edition, Johns Hopkins University Press.

Schaarschmidt, T. (2018). Ich Bin Nicht Verrückt, Ich Bin Revoluzzer! Antipsychiatrie. *Zeit*. http://www.zeit.de/wissen/gesundheit/2018-01/antipsychiatrie-psychiatrien-psychologie-patienten

Schneider, I. (1987). The Theory and Practice of Movie Psychiatry. *The American Journal of Psychiatry*, 144(8), 996–1002.

Schwager, M. (2012). Smearing the Medieval: Architectural Objects and Time Travel in Amnesia: The Dark Descent. *The Year's Work in Medievalism* 27. https://medievalists.net/2014/03/smearing-medieval-architectural-objects-time-travel-amnesia-dark-descent

Shelve, M. (2019). “Her Temper Was Still the Same”: Women Resisting Colonialism in Modern Viking Narratives. *The Heroic Age* 19. https://heroicage.net/issues/19/sheble.php

Simond, S. H. (in press). *Pixelated Madness. The Construction of Mental Ilnesses and Psychiatric Institutions in Video Games*. Verlag Werner Hülsbusch.

Therrien, C. (2009). Games of Fear: A Multi-Faceted Historical Account of the Horror Genre in Video Games. *Horror Video Games: Essays on the Fusion of Fear and Play*, 26–45.

Thon, J.-N. (2021). Playing with Fear: The Aesthetics of Horror in Recent Indie Games. *Eludamos: Journal for Computer Game Culture*, 10(1), 197–231.

Vozaru, M. (2022). Reclaiming Agency. Engaging Non-Human Agency for a Nuanced Portrayal of Mental Distress and Recovery. In Jimena Aguilar Rodríguez et al. (Eds.), *Mental Health | Atmospheres | Video Games. New Directions in Game Research II*, 63–76. transcript.

Wampold, B. E. (2001). Contextualizing Psychotherapy as a Healing Practice: Culture, History, and Methods. *Applied and Preventive Psychology* 10(2), 69–86.

## Referenced Games

AMNESIA: A MACHINE FOR PIGS. The Chinese Room, 2013.

AMNESIA: REBIRTH. Frictional Games, 2020.

AMNESIA: THE BUNKER. Frictional Games, 2023.

AMNESIA: THE DARK DESCENT. Frictional Games, 2010.

CALL OF CTHULHU. Chaosium, 1981.

CALL OF CTHULHU. Cyanide, Focus Entertainment, 2018.

CALL OF CTHULHU: DARK CORNERS OF THE EARTH. Headfirst Productions, Ubisoft, 2005.

CRUSADER KINGS III. Paradox Development Studio, 2020.

DARKEST DUNGEON. Red Hook Studios, 2016.

DMC: DEVIL MAY CRY. Ninja Theory, 2013.

DON'T STARVE. Klei Entertainment, 2013.

ENSLAVED: ODYSSEY TO THE WEST. Ninja Theory, 2010.

ETERNAL DARKNESS: SANITY'S REQUIEM. Silicon Knights, Nintendo, 2002.

HEAVENLY SWORD. Ninja Theory, 2007.

HELLBLADE: SENUA'S SACRIFICE. Ninja Theory, 2017.

INDIGO PROPHECY (FAHRENHEIT). Quantic Dream, 2005.

SENUA'S SAGA: HELLBLADE II. Ninja Theory, 2024.

THE SIMS 4. Maxis, 2014.

TOKYO DARK. Cherrymochi, Unties, 2017.

TOKYO DARK: REMEMBRANCE. Cherrymochi, Unties, 2019.

# Design Perspectives

# Lie in My Heart

## Designing an Autobiographical Expressive Game Exploring Suicide and Resilience

*Sébastien Genvo*

In the early 2010s, I began to work on the concept of expressive games as part of my research. It arose from an observation shared by a number of researchers and game designers in the 2000s. In the history of video games, certain themes have been overrepresented (e.g. science fiction, medieval fantasy, sport, war, Nordic or Asian myths, etc.), which has gone hand in hand with the dominant presence of certain emotions: anxiety, fear, anger. This is shown by Kline, Dyer Witheford and De Peuter (2003) in their book DIGITAL PLAY. For marketing, technological and cultural reasons, themes of "militarised masculinities" have spread in the industry's productions. According to these authors, this refers to an interrelation of ingredients that make up a shared semiotic network revolving around the subjects of war, conquest and combat. This dominant model has been tried and tested in the video game market, although it is very often the subject of debate and limits openness to other types of audiences. Gonzalo Frasca (2001) also put forward this idea in the very first issue of GAMESTUDIES.ORG, in an article about THE SIMS (Electronic Arts, 2000). Here he argues that video games should be opened up to realities that are more in tune with everyday life: "THE SIMS is a landmark in videogame history because it has opened a Pandora's box by replacing the usual troll and sci-fi monster with plain humans" (Frasca 2001).

What is interesting about Gonzalo Frasca's work is that he envisaged solutions. In particular, he considered that video games could be used as a medium to stimulate critical thinking about personal and social problems. In his work in the early 2000s, Gonzalo Frasca proposed drawing on the dramatic techniques of the Theatre of the Oppressed, introduced by Augusto Boal, in order to design games that encourage debate among players (see Frasca, 2001). To sum up very briefly, the Theatre of the Oppressed stages a situation of oppression during which any spectator can choose to intervene to take the place of a protagonist and propose their own solution to the problem. Frasca's aim was to show how the Theatre of the Oppressed philosophy could be applied to video games in order to increase its potential for raising awareness. In his view, this could encourage a logic of empathy based on the manipulation of rules and choices.

As part of these reflections, in the early 2010s I proposed the term "expressive game" (Genvo, 2016) to describe games that involve putting yourself in someone else's shoes to explore social, cultural or psychological issues, etc., while allowing you to experience the dilemmas, choices and consequences that arise from these situations. Firstly, the idea was to find a concept that could be used as an analytical framework for identifying this type of game in the history of video games. Indeed, in the history of this medium, there is some content that proposes alternative themes, albeit on the margins. Take, for example, the French productions of the 1980s, some of which were aimed at a local market and drew on cultural references relating to the current events of the period, or even to French history. The game FREEDOM (Tomahawk, 1988), published in 1988, tackled the history of slavery in Martinique by putting us in the shoes of a slave trying to escape from the plantations.

But it is also worth noting that studying the expressive potential of video games raises a number of questions, both from a creative and a scientific point of view: how can these works be considered as games, when they challenge the usual expectations associated with video games because of their sensitive subject matter? Games, particularly in the video game industry, are synonymous with fun and entertainment in today's society. How can we get players emotionally involved while at the same time encouraging them to reflect on the sensitive content developed in these games? And how could we build an experience which also allows a degree of expressivity from the player? It is from this dual perspective that I have been exploring the concept since 2010, both by exploring it in greater depth conceptually and by designing two games. KEYS OF A GAMESPACE (KOAG) (Expressive Gamestudio, 2011), designed in 2011, tackles the subject of child abuse and memory, and LIE IN MY HEART (LIMH) (Expressive Gamestudio, 2019) in 2019 takes an autobiographical approach to the themes of suicide, mental illness, the relationship between childhood and death, and resilience. The aim was to combine research and authorial work, which enables experimental objects to be designed and produced in order to test certain concepts.

To illustrate these theoretical considerations, I will show how this research is also anchored in a game design perspective, which prompts reflection. I will discuss the development of my game LIE IN MY HEART (2019). By doing so, I will explore how an individual life story can be shared. Surely there must be a contradiction in wanting to transmit a memory of established events while at the same time providing players with a form of agency to intervene in past events? More precisely, I will discuss the design choices that were made to encourage empathy and reflection on the multiple topics conveyed by the game. I will also look at the reception, particularly the emotional experience of the players and the way in which they were able to find and express themselves on the addressed topics. This feedback is based on press reviews, players' reviews on Steam and a qualitative analysis carried out with a dozen players. Finally, these perspectives will allow me to consider the personal experience evoked by the design of such an autobiographical game, which invites to both narrate and play with the self, oscillating between narrativity of the past and agency. The aim is to show that sublimating experience through creation does not necessarily lead to improved psychological well-being for the creator. Through the mediation of experience, it more certainly enables the construction of a shareable meaning of the past.

## Imagining video game expressiveness beyond procedural rhetoric

In the early 2010s, when I was beginning to formalise the concept of expressive games, one of the main references directly addressing the question of the expressivity of video games was Ian Bogost's (2007) PERSUASIVE GAMES: THE EXPRESSIVE POWER OF VIDEOGAMES. Following in the footsteps of Frasca, with whom he has collaborated on several projects,[1] Bogost argues that for video games to count as expressive artefacts, it is necessary to understand how they can be designed to support arguments about the way our world works. Bogost argues that video games give form to a new sort of rhetoric, which he calls procedural rhetoric. Video games can persuade others based on a system of rules. The point of view developed by Ian Bogost is similar to that of Frasca (2003), for whom video games are to be understood as forms of simulation. While Bogost stresses that procedurality can be found outside computer systems (it can be found in the courts, in bureaucracy etc.), it nevertheless distinguishes computers from other media, because the computer makes intensive use of it. For Bogost, it is necessary to study procedural rhetoric in order to better analyse, criticise and even design "persuasive games". These are particular types of video games that seek to make the user adhere to the content of a discourse based on procedures.

However, exploring the expressive potential of video games cannot be approached solely through issues of persuasion. This is partly what Frasca's early work hinted at, showing that it is possible to think of video games as a way of sharing a problematic life experience, without necessarily wishing to convince people of a pre-established solution. To understand what an "expressive" (and not just "persuasive") video game would be—one that would express a social or psychological problem, etc., to the player and at the same time allow them to express themselves around the issue—requires to take into account that expressiveness comes both from the procedures induced by the structure of the game and from the actions

1 In 2003, for example, they worked together on HOWARD DEAN FOR IOWA, which was the first official video game for a US presidential candidate, aimed at convincing voters to vote for that candidate in the Democratic primaries.

carried out by the player. This is a criticism that has already been levelled at Bogost's approach, as it overlooks the player's role in the process. According to Miguel Sicart (2011), the message conveyed by a game should be seen as a conversation between the game and the players, who have their own beliefs and values. In my opinion, this also applies to the perception of what is or isn't a game: each player has their own idea of what a game is, depending on their cultural context, their biographical journey as a player, and their skills. In short, to use one of Bogost's definitions of rhetoric, my rhetorical approach to defining "expressive" games seeks to understand the processes that establish "the effective arrangement of a work so as to create a desirable possibility space for interpretation" (Bogost 2007, p. 20). In other words, one of the main concerns in designing an expressive game is to enable the player to recognise themselves by allowing them to play on the values conveyed by the game. It is a question of implementing a certain form of agency in the solutions proposed so that the players can recognise themselves in some way. The intention is to get them to think about the situations presented while at the same time involving them emotionally, in particular by developing empathy. In short, compared with persuasive games, the aim of expressive games is to take a broader approach to expressiveness. Games can also express a point of view on complex societal issues and can encourage public debate without prescribing certain messages and values.

In this context, a reflection on the expressive specificities of video games must take into account what constitutes their ludic dimension, which is often forgotten in research on the subject. Procedurality and simulation are part of video games, but not all procedures and simulations are considered to be games. My research is based in particular on the observation that, in order to become meaningful, games must be considered by the player as an intermediate area of experience between reality and fiction, based on the theories of play and fantasy developed by the child psychiatrist D.W. Winnicott. For Winnicott (1971), the area of play is not inner psychic reality. It is outside the individual, but it is not the external world. While the chess player is meticulous in moving each of their pieces while considering the consequences of their decisions, their gesture cannot be summed up in this action alone. As chess fans say, it is not just a matter of "pushing wood". To really enter the game, the player must "pretend" that the board and the pieces are more than just what they are, but without taking the "simulacra" for reality; the player must enter into a universe of singular meaning. They will transpose the things of the world in which they live into a new order, governed both by the rules of everyday life and by rules specific to the game. But the player is not totally abstracted from "ordinary reality" either; playing is not dreaming. In short, to get someone to play and consider an object or situation as a game, they need to enter this intermediate area of experience, between reality and fiction. These ways of sharing meaningful play (Salen and Zimmerman, 2004) is what I call a process of ludic mediation.

Therefore, for a game to be genuinely considered as such and induce a state of play, it has to proceed to what I call a "ludic mediation": designing a game requires an understanding of the modalities of transmission of a shared meaning of play. This approach to games can be found in Bateson's (1977) theories of play, who stressed that play is an act of communication, based on the exchange of messages or signals. From this perspective, it can be argued that gaming-oriented devices try to convince the recipient of their playfulness by meeting certain cultural representations of the activity. By doing so, games also convey a system of values that depict a given representation of what a game is. Questioning the expressive scope of games therefore also means asking what system of values a game expresses and how it is possible to enable players to find their way around it, to recognise themselves in it, so that it corresponds to their idea of what a game is.

To illustrate these theoretical considerations, I will demonstrate how they formed the basis of my latest research-creation project and the way the game was received.

## Lie in my Heart: Expressive games as an act of autobiographical testimony

It should be pointed out that, in video games in general, the autobiographical form is hardly developed at all, even though this genre is common in other media. This lack of autobiographical games can perhaps be explained by the usual association of games with a form of agency: players want to have the feeling that they have choices and that their actions have significant repercussions. How can this be reconciled with conveying a series of pre-established biographical facts? This is the question posed by the few existing biographical games. THAT DRAGON, CANCER (Numinous Games, 2016), for example, tells the story of its creator's experience of his newborn baby's cancer. To stay within the framework of a game, a number of metaphorical scenes are used, in line with the more general perspective described by Doris C. Rusch (2017), when dealing with feelings about life issues in games. The use of metaphor is a way of encouraging players not to place themselves solely on the side of the reality of a situation, which would not allow them to enter the intermediate area of experience referred to by D.W. Winnicott. However, in terms of agency, THAT DRAGON, CANCER has chosen to constrain the player by leaving them little latitude as to how the events unfold.

The question of biography in video games is therefore a particularly stimulating one for exploring the specific features of games as a means of expression. They raise the question of how it is possible to reconcile agency with the imperatives of testimony, while allowing the player to find their way beyond an individual experience that is firmly rooted in reality (all the more so if the theme is traumatic). I recently explored the subject in the development of LIE IN MY HEART (LIMH). In this visual novel, the player discovers a series of events that affected me a few years ago. My son's mother, named Marie in the game, decided to take her own life. Among other things, she suffered from bipolar disorder, although her decision to end her life cannot be summed up in terms of these disorders. Beyond the experience of this individual tragedy and the questioning of its causes, there are also questions about how to support the child through this event, and about resilience. One of the first ways of reconciling agency with the biographical dimension was to draw on counterfactual history (Deluermoz and Sinagaravélou, 2016). This is a form of historical approach that allows the exploration of alternative and probable scenarios in order to better understand the factors that influence the course of a series of events. This seemed particularly appropriate to the issue of questioning the causes of the tragedy, which is one of the central points of the experiment. One of the methodological recommendations of counterfactual history is to encourage comparison between the alternative scenario and the actual event.

It is this approach that has been developed in LIMH and which, in my opinion, has enabled me to go beyond the tension between testimony and agency: the players are free to follow their own path through alternative scenarios, but at the end of each sequence a commentary tells them how many of the choices they have made are identical to those made in the "real world". However, the player is not told which choices were identical, in order to encourage replayability (it takes around 1 hr 30 min to complete the game). At the end of the first game, players are given a clue to help them identify the choices that correspond to the real world. Players can then try to bridge the gap between their choices and those in the biographical itinerary in a later game. This was also intended to allow the player to adopt a more reflective attitude, after an initial experience that was more oriented towards emotional and empathic involvement. In this way, the game constantly oscillates between a certain autobiographical form, closer to reality, and an autofictional form, departing from past events through the player's choices, which constitutes an intermediate area of experience conducive to play. As the game is a visual novel, there is a point to be made about its gameplay, which may seem minimalist given the game's genre. This may run counter to the sense of agency that players expect to encounter, and may question their perception of LIMH as a game. However, for me (Genvo, 2009), gameplay should be defined as the space of possibilities that the game offers and that the player is given to actualise in his action. In this respect, even if it is minimalist, the gameplay here is enriched by the choices left to the player and his confrontation with the various other possibilities, based on an approach nourished by counterfactual history.

From this perspective, one of the design choices was therefore to allow the player to have an impact on the course of certain events, but above all to allow them to express their own values in response to the events presented, which is not the approach taken in biographical video games up to now. For example, in THAT DRAGON, CANCER, the tragedy we are presented with—a father's experience of his newborn baby with cancer—is approached through the prism of a Christian vision of death, which helped the designer overcome the tragedy. In LIE IN MY HEART, the choice was made to leave the player free to explain death to the child according to different value systems (believers or non-believers). Later, if they wish, the player can discover how the death was really explained.

In this way, the expressiveness of the game is as much that of the work as that of the player, even if the latter is always limited. The difficulty lies in deciding which scenes or elements should be restricted and which should be left to the player to choose from. As a designer, the question was to know how much to open up the possibilities of choice in certain scenes (and what choices to give the player), while at the same time respecting the narrative that you want to convey, so that it remains consistent with what you want to show. The choice has been made, however, to always adjust the dialogue in one way or another according to the player's actions, a sometimes subtle adjustment that does not completely disrupt certain key events in the plot.

On the other hand, in order to reinforce the testimonial dimension of the game, another atypical choice compared with biographical games was to move away from a metaphorical approach to the situations presented, which strongly distinguishes LIMH from other productions of this type. The fact that the game is more firmly rooted in real-life events is reflected in the artistic direction. "Marie" was an artist, for example, and some of her paintings or art installations were included in several scenes, sometimes directly in photographs as an open window onto the past and reality, or sometimes as an interactive element offering gameplay features. Several scenes in the game are also taken from photographs taken during our life as a couple. However, as I have argued above, in order to play, an individual must consider a situation as an intermediate area of experience, between reality and fiction. The risk of this highly reality-based approach was that it would be very difficult to see the experience as a game, especially given the topic we were tackling. To develop the playful dimension, each scene was reworked by superimposing pencil drawings and digital painting, turning the different sequences into intermediate areas between reality and fiction.

Similarly, some of the characters (a policeman, a journalist, etc.) are caricatures of other fictional characters. This gives a particular connotation to the scene for the players, who can pick up on the reference. This opens up a form of semiotic contingency (to use a term developed by Malaby, 2007), with interpretative playability in the meaning of certain scenes. There is for instance a police inspector whose name and features are reminiscent of the French comedian Coluche in the film INSPECTEUR LA BAVURE (Zidi, 1980). In a way, these caricatured references inscribe LIE IN MY HEART within a specific ludic culture: that of the French adventure games of the

1980s, where it was not uncommon to come across references to the audiovisual, cinematographic, musical, and even political landscape of France at the time.

*Figures 1: (top) and 2 (bottom): Screenshots from LIMH. The images are a combination of sketches and photographs*

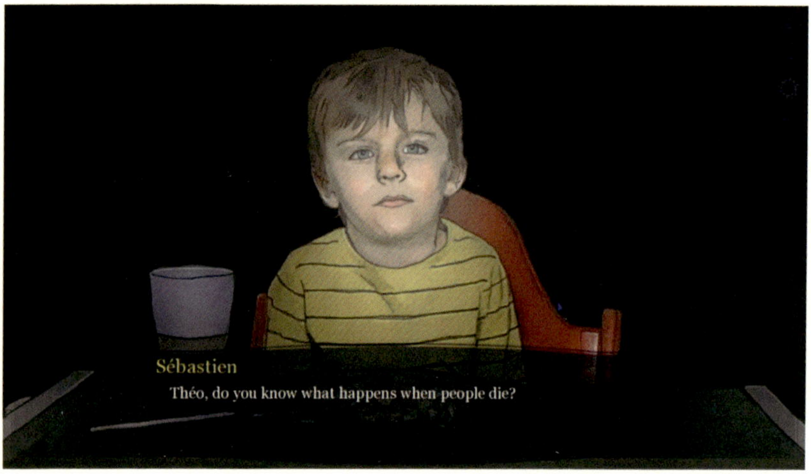
Sébastien
Théo, do you know what happens when people die?

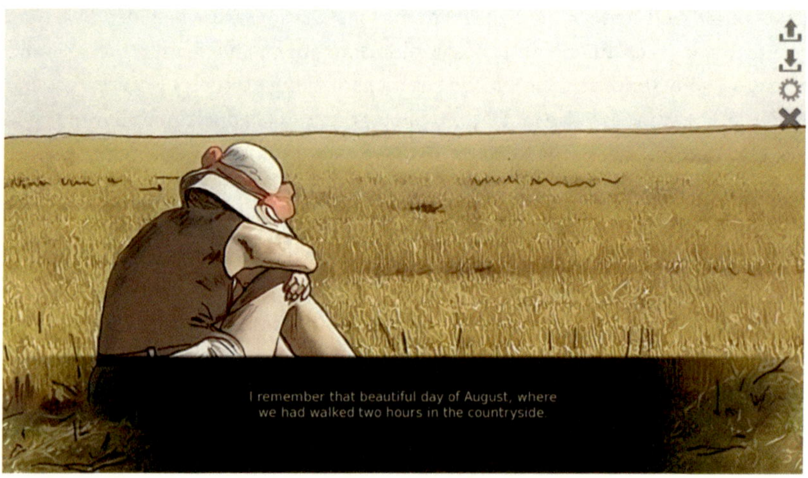
I remember that beautiful day of August, where
we had walked two hours in the countryside.

The game LE DOSSIER BOERHAAVE (Infogrames, 1987) comes to mind, where the player leads a police investigation around the Père Lachaise cemetery, encountering caricatures of Jacques Chirac. LIE IN MY HEART is also set in a local area, with several elements indicating that the events take place in Louvigny, a village in eastern France where Marie and I lived. In my opinion, these culturally rooted references further reinforce the sense of reality conveyed by certain aspects of the game. However, the fact that the game is rooted in a specific ludic culture and a precise locality raises the question of ludic mediation on an intercultural scale (especially as the game is distributed on Steam and available in English), hence the importance of implementing game mechanisms that allow players to recognise themselves.

Regarding the reception of the game, several sources provided feedback on the various theoretical and design choices developed in LIMH. Before the game was distributed on Steam, an initial qualitative analysis was carried out on 8 French players (4 men and 4 women) of different ages (from 21 to 62) and with different levels of skill (from regular to very occasional players). The aim was to explore the players' emotional feelings after a gaming session (by helping them to verbalise their feelings using the Geneva Emotion Wheel) (Scherer et al., 2013), as well as their reflections on the topics covered, and their perception of the ludic dimension of the work (is it a game?). The players were interviewed directly after a game session. The interviews were conducted using a grid of semi-directive questions based on a final version of the game. For the recruitment, none of the players knew me personally or my work in progress, in order to ensure a fresh and neutral view of the story. The interviews were conducted by a third party in my absence. These initial analyses confirmed the strong emotional charge that the game could carry, with almost all of the subjects (7/8) stating that they had felt strong emotions, such as sadness (6/8), compassion (4/8), anger (5/8, particularly with regard to the feeling of powerlessness over certain events), and joy (4/8, particularly with regard to the poetic ending or some happy memories). As for the reflective aspect, a large majority (6/8) said that the game prompted them to ask questions, to reflect or to want to find out more about the issues they had identified (mental illness, suicide, relationship problems, children's experience of difficult situations). More generally, all the players (8/8) said that they were familiar with the story and recognised themselves in it, whether in terms of the situations described or the characters (whether the character of Sébastien, Marie, or even the child). This endorsement tends to validate the theoretical and design choices that were made to enable players to "recognise themselves" in the game, by allowing the player to express themself while maintaining a logic of biographical testimony. What's more, when we asked the players why they recognised themselves in the game, many of them immediately spoke about their own personal experiences. Two of the players in the sample, for example, said they had experienced the suicide of someone close to them or had felt suicidal themselves. This suggests that expressive games can help people to talk about traumatic experiences.

It should be noted that this involvement of players in the storyline was also reflected in the reviews left on LIMH's steam page following the game's release.[2] This provided another source for analysing the reception of the game beyond the initial qualitative analyses. These reviews highlighted the possibility of anchoring a story locally while reaching players from a variety of cultural backgrounds, which was one of the questions at the heart of the design choices. For example, positive reviews from players of different nationalities (including Russians and Chinese) emphasised the emotional impact of the game ("The end result moved me in a way I don't think a game has ever moved me before"), as well as the identification dimension that certain aspects of the game allow, as one Russian player put it: "The game is designed so that the player is SEBASTIEN and that we see him in his role. That's what the game is all about—so that we put on a person's mask and can see events on their behalf".

The empathic and emotional aspect, already identified by the qualitative analyses, is also found in press articles. The newspaper Le Parisien stated, for example, that "Sébastien Genvo has designed an autobiographical video game in which he invites the player to reflect on emotions such as sadness and empathy" (Henry, 2019). This is also true of the reflexive dimension of the experience. This is the case, for example, in an article about LIMH in the newspaper Le Monde: "The use of video games as a medium is not insignificant: it allows us to question the uncertain degree of control we believe we have over our own lives and those of our loved ones" (Audureau, 2019). A similar comment was made by Eurogamer.com, which described the alternation between engagement and distancing that gamers can experience: "The different paths created by Genvo are fascinating. While playing, you'll find yourself instinctively leaning in certain directions, then questioning whether you should have gone that way" (Allen, 2019). But whether it is in the qualitative analysis, the players' reviews or the press, all the sources contain discussions about LIMH's status as a game.

The Eurogamer.com article begins as follows: "Lie in my Heart isn't really a game. OK, it is technically, but it's also the story of an awful time in one man's life" (Allen, 2019). Some of the players' attempts at definition tend to bring it closer to more classic narrative forms. For example, a player on Steam described it as a diary: "More than a game, it's an extract from a diary, a slice of life that hurts". Other players emphasise the atypical emotional aspect for a video game: "This game was so moving for me that I found it hard to define it as such. It's a real experience that can make you learn about yourself and make you think about complex situations". Several players in the qualitative survey also emphasised the fact that this experience was a departure from traditional forms of gaming. For example, one of the participants pointed out that a game should normally take the individual away from reality, while another said that a game is supposed to be joyful. We can see that the connotations conferred

2 https://store.steampowered.com/app/1116490/Lie_In_My_Heart/

on what a game is strongly structure the experience of some players, leading them to question whether it really is a game at all. Other players, however, show in their opinions that this questioning has led them to redefine their expectations in terms of games. This shows that questioning the ludic status of an "atypical" work can lead individuals to change their own representations of what a game is, as shown by this player's opinion on Steam: "You could even say that it paves the way for a new genre of video games; autobiographical games, even memorial games. It's more than just a Visual Novel, it's an experience, where you put yourself in the author's shoes, make choices, then ask yourself questions and step back to reflect…". This is also the meaning of the conclusion of an article in the newspaper Libération: "Lie in My Heart's greatest contribution may simply be to broaden the scope of what video games can be" (Chapuis, 2019). This comment in a national daily newspaper for the wider public shows that opening up games to new expressive horizons is now likely to appeal to a wide audience. It also shows that questioning the expressiveness of video games is a way of exploring new creative horizons.

## Experiencing the process of creation

While this article has developed the scientific motivations behind the project, I would like to conclude by returning to the motivations behind the creative process as such and the personal experiences associated with it. This kind of reflexive feedback has yet to be extensively documented in the context of the creation of an autobiographical game,[3] even though the nature of the project is particularly stimulating in terms of self-reflection. In my opinion, this approach can make a contribution both scientifically and creatively. In recent years, the release of LIMH has led me to give a large number of talks to a wide variety of audiences, including academic conferences on the concept of expressive games, talks as part of art exhibitions (for example, the game was exhibited in May and June 2023 at the National Centre for the Arts in Mexico) and talks at health-related events (for example, in 2023 I gave a talk to an association concerned with the issue of bipolar disorders). A recurring question from the audience at these various events concerns the effects of making such a game on my own experience and feelings about the past events (a question I have also been asked by the editors of this book). These questions often raise the public's hypothesis of the cathartic dimension of such a creation, which would lead to the development of a form of resilience or facilitate healing with regard to the wounds of the past.

---

3 I should mention the documentary THANK YOU FOR PLAYING (Osit, Zouhali-Worrall, 2015), which looks back at the process of creating the game THAT DRAGON, CANCER (Numinous Games, 2016).

The answer I usually give is that I didn't start designing the game until I had already put some distance between myself and the emotional charge of the past (the events took place in 2017 and I started designing at the end of 2018). So I didn't need to create this game to be able to work through my grief or to begin the process of resilience. On the contrary, creating the game required me to delve back into this experience to reconstruct certain events or to envisage probable alternatives, in order to imagine the choices left to the player. In this sense, it would have been easier to develop my resilience if I had not been engaged in the creation of the game, especially as its existence and the role played by this game in my professional activity continue to render these past events present. Nevertheless, I also say in response that one of the reasons that led me to design this game is to help build and give shared meaning to these events. For me, art is a way of reflecting on ourselves, on others and on the world around us, while at the same time being touched emotionally. It is this perspective of artistic creation that has guided me above all, aiming to share with the players an emotion of "extimising empathy", as the psychiatrist Serge Tisseron (2011) puts it. This is a form of empathy that enables us to put ourselves in the other person's shoes, to discover that we are different from what we thought we were, and to allow ourselves to be transformed by this discovery. It was this kind of extimising empathy that *Lie in my Heart* was aiming for. That empathy is reflected in the feedback of some of the players on Steam, who talk about the impact the game has had on their own lives. A French player says: "This game has had an impact on me and is playing a role in my current situation... I can easily identify with Marie, and I'm thinking of reviewing some of the decisions I've made about my health as a result of this experience. So thank you..."

My experience and my intention with regard to creation are largely in line with Eloisa Castellano-Maury's (2014) reflections on the boundaries of sublimation between creativity and creation. Referring to Freud's concept of sublimation, she indicates that it concerns human activities detached from pulsion and directed towards cultural objectives valued by society. In this category, at the end of a successful psychoanalytic treatment, would be creativity, i.e. an achievement that belongs to what can be called the "small sublimations". Creativity can be a favourable factor in the life of a subject freed from his neurotic inhibitions by analysis, and who can now devote themself to activities that will bring real satisfaction. However, according to this author, creations do not fall into this sublimatory category. Creation may have little or nothing to do with the analytical treatment and does not necessarily lead to recovery or a better psychological balance. Creation takes a longer route. For Eloisa Castellano-Maury, what characterises creation above all is its "innovative" aspect. It takes the form of completely new and original works, which distinguishes it from creativity. In this respect, she takes the example of several artists for whom creation was not synonymous with psychic healing (Verlaine, Proust, Bacon, etc.).

In a sense, this demonstration also echoes D.W. Winnicott's comments on the boundary between creativity and creation. For this child psychiatrist, the intermediate area of experience constituted by play is first and foremost an area where the baby can experience the process of separation from the mother without it being traumatic. For Winnicott, in this context, the question of separation does not arise because, in the potential space between mother and baby, a "creative play" arises quite naturally from the state of relaxation. It is through this creativity, enabled by play, that the baby can glimpse a new way of being in the world, separated from the mother. In this respect, Donald W. Winnicott goes so far as to consider that it is through play, and only through play, that the individual, whether child or adult, is capable of being creative and using their entire personality. For him, creativity is understood as the colouring of a whole attitude towards external reality. But it is also important to emphasise that this creativity can then permeate every moment of life, be present in everyday life, and not just in artistic creation. Winnicott (1988) insists on distinguishing between creative living and artistic creation. For him, living creatively is deeply linked to the feeling that you are alive and yourself. But he distinguishes this from a work of creation, which he sees first and foremost as the establishment of a shared reality. For him, the work of creation lies between the receiver and the artist's creativity.[4]

All of these reflections are ultimately in line with my own experience of the creation process. The creativity that goes into creating a work or playing a game can be a way of expressing our personality and having moments where we feel alive. But in itself, LIE IN MY HEART was intended to create an intermediate area of experience between my own experience and that of the player, who will also be able to express their creativity to a certain extent when playing. While this creation does not necessarily provide a form of healing for the author (that was not the aim of the creation and I did not embark on the project with this intention in mind), it does provide a space for creativity aimed at co-constructing a new, unprecedented meaning through the interweaving of several experiences, my own and those of the players. In short, by creating LIE IN MY HEART, the aim was to keep the memory of a past still alive through the games of the players. This is one of the reasons why the game closes with an extract from Lord Tennyson's poem, which I will also quote here to conclude this text:

"Never, oh! never,
nothing will die;
The stream flows,
The wind blows,
The cloud fleets,

4 For an in-depth analysis of Winnicott's work on creation and creativity, see Aubourg (2003).

The heart beats,
Nothing will die."

## References


Allen, J. (2019). Lie in My Heart and Dealing with the Aftermath. *Eurogamer.* https://www.eurogamer.net/articles/2019-11-13-lie-in-my-heart-and-dealing-with-the-aftermath

Aubourg, F. (2003). Winnicott et la Créativité. *Le Coq-Héron* 173(2).

Audureau, W. (2019). Lie in My Heart, Jeu Vidéo Poignant sur les Thèmes du Suicide et du Deuil. *LeMonde.* https://www.lemonde.fr/pixels/article/2019/10/07/lie-in-my-heart-jeu-video-poignant-sur-les-themes-du-suicide-et-du-deuil_6014505_4408996.html

Bateson, G. (1977). *Vers une Ecologie de L'Esprit*. Paris : Seuil.

Bogost, I. (2007). *Persuasive Games: The Expressive Power of Video Games*. Cambridge, MA: MIT Press.

Castellano-Maury, E. (2014). Frontières de la Sublimation entre Créativité et Création. *Revue Française de Psychosomatique*, 46, 103–114.

Chapuis, M. (2019). Lie in My Heart, Niveaux de Vie. *Libération.* https://next.liberation.fr/images/2019/10/25/lie-in-my-heart-niveaux-de-vie_1759735

Deluermoz, Q., Sinagaravélou, P. (2016). *Pour une Histoire des Possibles: Analyses Contrefactuelles et Futurs Non Advenus*. Paris : Le Seuil.

Expressive Gamestudio (2011). KEYS OF A GAMESPACE. Expressive Gamestudio.

Expressive Gamestudio (2019). LIE IN MY HEART. Cogaming Rising.

Frasca, G. (2001). The Sims: Grandmothers are Cooler than Trolls. *Game Studies* 1. http://www.gamestudies.org/0101/frasca/

Frasca, G. (2003). Simulation versus Narrative. In Mark J. P. Wolf and Bernard Perron (Eds.), *The Video Game Theory Reader*. New York: Routledge.

Genvo, S. (2009). *Le Jeu à Son Ère Numérique: Comprendre et Analyser les Jeux Vidéo*. L'Harmattan.

Genvo, S. (2016). Defining and Designing Expressive Games: The Case of Keys of a Gamespace. *Kinephanos Journal of Media Studies and Popular Culture*, Special Issue April 2016, https://www.kinephanos.ca/2016/defining-and-designing-expressive-games/

Henry, D. (2019). Un chercheur lorraine crée un jeu vidéo sur le deuil. *Le Parisien*. https://www.leparisien.fr/high-tech/un-chercheur-lorrain-cree-un-jeu-video-sur-le-deuil-10-10-2019-8169945.php

Infogrames (1987). DOSSIER BOERHAAVE. Infogrames.

Kline, S. Dyer-Witheford, N. and De Peuter, G. (2003). Digital Play. The Interaction of Technology, Culture, and Marketing. Montreal & Kingston: McGill-Queen's University Press.

Malaby, T. M. (2007). Beyond Play. A New Approach to Games. *Games and Culture* 2(2), 95–113.

Maxis (2000). THE SIMS. Electronic Arts.

Numinous Games (2016). THAT DRAGON, CANCER. Numinous games.

Rusch, D. C. (2017). *Making Deep Games.* New York: CRC Press.

Salen K., Zimmerman E. (2004). *Rules of Play. Game Design Fundamentals*. Cambridge, MA: MIT Press.

Scherer, K.R., Shuman, V., Fontaine. J. R. J. and Soriano, C. (2013). The Grid Meets the Wheel: Assessing Emotional Feeling via Self-Report. In R. J. J. Fontaine, R. Klaus Scherer and C. Soriano (Eds.), *Components of Emotinoal Meaning: A Sourcebook*, 281–298. Oxford: Oxford University Press.

Sicart, M. (2011). Against Procedurality. *Game Studies* 11(3). http://gamestudies.org/1103/articles/sicart_ap

Tisseron, S. & Bass, H. (2011). L'Empathie au coeur du jeu social. *Le Journal des Psychologues*, 286, 20–23.

Tomahawk (1988). FREEDOM: LES GUERRIERS DE L'OMBRE. Coktel Vision.

Winnicott, D. W. (1971). *Jeu et Realite, L'Espace Potentiel*. Paris: Gallimard.

Winnicott, D. W. (1988). *Vivre Créativement. Conversations Ordinaires.* Paris, Gallimard.

Zidi, C. (1980). *Inspecteur la Bavure.* France.

# Colorful Depression

## How to Create a Bright Game about a Dark Topic

*Kerstin Schütt*

Depression. The word alone has for many an uncomfortable weight. That barrier makes it hard to learn about the topic, despite depression being one of the more common mental disorders. According to the WHO, approximately 280 million people in the world have depression and more than 700,000 die through suicide, making it a life-threatening mental disorder (WHO, 2023). Knowing this does not make the weight that the word alone holds any lighter. But this circumstance was one of the mayor inspirations why we, Twisted Ramble Games, created DURU: A colourful game about depression. And mole rats.

On the following pages, I will share our method of creating a light-hearted game about a dark topic. First I offer a brief description of the game and the goals we set for ourselves. Afterwards you get a step-by-step approach for creating such a game yourself, and I share some pitfalls to look out for when dealing with sensitive subject matter. At the end I discuss briefly the potential that these kinds of games hold and what we learned while creating one.

### What is *Duru – About Mole Rats and Depression*?

At its heart, DURU is a 2D puzzle platformer set in a colourful, West African-inspired mole rat colony. Players experience the game as Tuli, a food gatherer of the colony who also loves painting and enjoying life with her mole rat friends. While she is small in stature, she is very agile and has the magical ability to draw objects from her mind into reality. Thus players are challenged to overcome obstacles in the tunnels surrounding the colony by running, jumping and painting their way through various obstacles on the lookout for food.

*Figure 1: Banner illustration for Duru's Steam page*

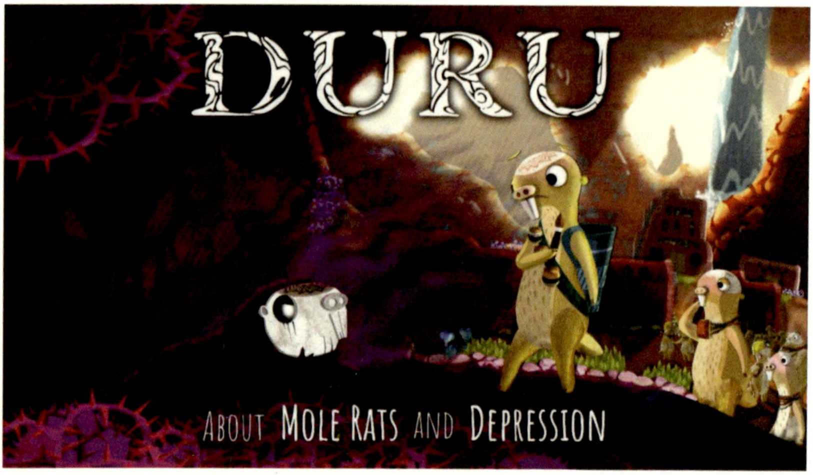


One day, life gets harder when the food storage of the colony is plagued by a maggot infestation, and everybody is encouraged by the mole rat queen to give 110%, a phrase that might be okay in the encouraging speech of a team coach in a sport movie but not in a work environment. Tuli finds herself lacking, thinking she underperforms when she really works harder than before. It is during this time that her life gets even more challenging when seemingly out of nowhere a dark, 6-legged creature joins her. It goes by the name of Bel and is an AI companion that follows Tuli everywhere. Bel manipulates objects that players paint into the world, holds Tuli back when she moves too far away and introduces a whole new puzzle element to players.

Bel can only be seen by Tuli and, of course, players, while it is invisible to the other mole rats. It does not only serve a purpose in terms of game mechanics but is also a narrative element: Bel manipulates Tuli's thoughts, making her think less of herself and puts all the bad thoughts into her mind when she is just about to fall asleep at night.

Duru, through its colourful art style, cute characters and intuitive gameplay, poses a low barrier towards the topic of depression. The word itself never even makes it into the game apart from the subtitle: all dialog is shown in the form of pictures, making it a more individual story since everybody interprets the dialog a little differently, a little bit more towards their own experiences. The game not only shows common symptoms of depression through story and mechanics, it also depicts common misconceptions other people share about it and their well-intended but sometimes involuntarily hurtful way of dealing with someone who suffers from this disorder. We did not only want to raise awareness about depression and the behaviours to avoid while interacting with someone afflicted by it, but also show little things everybody can do to help someone, like constantly reaching out even if there's no response and not shaming someone for cancelling last minute or for socially withdrawing. In short: DURU is a game to educate about depression and encourage further empathy.

## Twisted Ramble's step-by-step guide to creating colourful serious games

While working on DURU we created a little guide for ourselves and other game developers to go about creating a colourful game with a serious or dark topic. There are certainly other ways to do so but this is a good starting point, especially when it is your first time creating such a game. I will explain every step in detail, but at the end of this part, there is a little overview to refresh your memory when you want to come back to it.

The first step, of course, is gathering information. This one is true for other games as well when finding a setting or an art style. Both fields are not included in this step. Before you do anything else you want to know your topic. Even if it is one you yourself are affected by, you need to read up on it. Literally. While the internet is a vast pool of information, books are edited, curated and most of the time more reliable as a source of information. That counts double on topics like (mental) disorders, medical issues and historic conflicts.

Cooperations with institutes, organizations or NGOs will set you on a good path from the get-go but are harder to come by. It might be easier to find an expert you can talk with about the chosen topic. Often enough you can find a dedicated person among those experts and befriend them. Having someone to message a quick question to during your development process is invaluable.

During your research you should keep an extra file in which you collect hopeful or positive moments, things that helped people getting through the darkness. Those are the things you want in your colourful serious game!

After collecting your information, step two is to **define your game's goal**. I'm not talking about mechanics though. Why do you want to create a game about this topic in the first place, and what should players take away from it? Possible goals can be raising awareness, give voice to an inside perspective, explain something complicated in a playful way, give advice, etc.

Similar to this: when a character in your story has a mental disorder or a disability, ask yourself the question why. To depict the diverse world we live in is a good enough reason, it doesn't have to be fancy. Just keep in mind that disorders and disabilities are NOT character traits. In public perception are some myths around that: people with depression are "weak", people with anxiety are always shy, people with borderline personality disorder are "attention seekers". There is also a generalization of people with mental disorders being dangerous to others when quite the opposite is the case: people with a mental illness are ten times more likely to be the victim of a violent crime. (Hazel, 2019).

In many games, we see plenty of bad examples of those misconceptions and stereotypes. Many horror games take place in so-called asylums or have a section of it take place in one or a hospital.

Asylums are pretty much depicted as prisons for "crazy", violent people: OUTLAST (Red Barrels, 2013) is one example of that in which the patients have violently taken over the facility and try to murder the player character, an investigative journalist, in various brutal manners. For some reason nearly all the inmates are naked as well, as if an unhealthy state of mind leads directly to nudity.

The same goes for BATMAN: ARKHAM ASYLUM (Rocksteady Studios, 2019) and, if you think about it, the whole Batman franchise since many villains are portrait with some unspecified form of mental illness which fuels their violent behaviour.

In the BORDERLANDS franchise there is a "class" of enemies called "Psychos" that are standard enemies to attack the player and to be killed by them. In BORDERLANDS 2 there is a playable character called "Krieg" who belongs to the "psycho class". In his background story it is mentioned that he endured abuse by his mother, suggesting that that made him tough and violent himself.

A study that looked at 456 games found that 54 of those included a representation of a mental illness with 57 instances overall in these games. Out of those 75% were negative portrayals and only one instance could be viewed as positive (Buday et al., 2022).

So if you plan to create a game about a mental disorder or include a character with a mental disorder, don't make them violent because of their disorder. Make it your goal to break those misconceptions and stereotypes. As you see, it is desperately needed.

Armed with your knowledge and goals, you can move on to the next step: **translate your research into game mechanics and story.** The first might seem to be the trickiest bit. You can create a colourful serious game with only the story rooted in your topic. But I like to challenge you to take full advantage of the medium you're working with and find mechanics that represent your topic as well. Following are some things that might help you achieve that.

Try and find the most significant or most common things about your subject. Curate your research instead of trying to fit everything into one game. Keep your goal in mind as well. To make this step seem less abstract, let's look at DURU. The most common symptoms of depression we depict in our game are:

- Distorted thought patterns and perception
- Changes in appetite
- Feelings of excessive guilt
- Low self-worth, feeling like a burden, self-blame

- Social isolation
- Loss of interest in activities and hobbies
- Disturbed sleep patterns (WHO, 2023)

In addition to that, we found while gathering information about our topic that many described depression as "an outside force"[1]. Some described it as a shadow constantly looming over them, others as a kraken whose many arms will always entangle them in one way or another. We used this perception of the illness to create Bel. It also helps with our goal of furthering an understanding for the illness and dealing with misconceptions: depression is not "a character flaw", it is not something intrinsic to Tuli. It is an illness, something from the outside that makes easy things hard and manipulates thoughts. Whenever Tuli experiences distorted thought patterns, it is depicted in a way that shows they're coming from Bel. Tuli has a harder time at work because Bel is hindering her. She has to work harder than everybody else, thus being constantly exhausted.

*Figure 2: Tuli declines hanging out with her friend. We as players can see why*

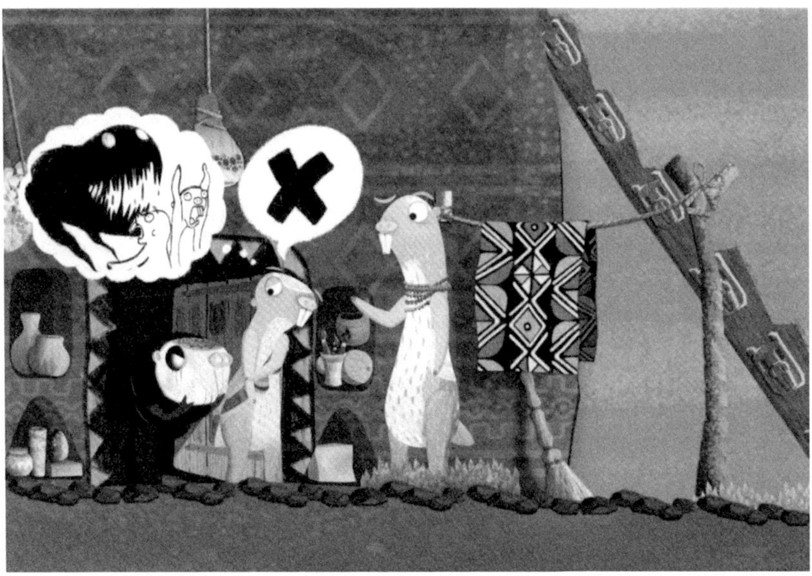

1 We gathered that information from personal experience, talks with friends with depression and from the amazing German project "Die Mitte der Nacht ist der Anfang vom Tag" which, among other things, gathers personal stories from afflicted persons. https://die-mitte-der-nacht.de/home

When Tuli can't participate in social activities, we as the player see it is because she thinks Bel might be a danger to others. In addition, when she thinks about talking to others about Bel, she is afraid of being called "crazy": saying that there is an invisible monster making her life harder and making her think bad things is a huge hurdle when no one else ever shared an experience like that.

When you look at the list of symptoms we picked, you will certainly find some missing. Especially the one that makes depression a life-threatening disease: suicide. When creating a colourful game about a dark topic, my advice is to avoid going to extremes if your game and message can be understood without it. This is why Tuli never expresses suicidal thoughts or self-harming behaviours in DURU.

If you can't find a game mechanic that translates your topic well, try to create one that emulates a feeling that matches what you are trying to convey. In addition to that, you can change the environment of the world or characters or even the sound and music.

With your gameplay and story in place, it's time for the last step: **make your game colourful**. Do you remember that extra file with the hopeful moments and positive experiences from your research? Now it's time for it to do your work. Include happy experiences or positive behaviours in your story and ideally in your gameplay as well. In DURU we do that by showing helpful behaviour of the other mole rats towards Tuli since one of our goals is to give advice not to people with depression, but to their immediate social circle. One friend of Tuli's visits her constantly and makes sure she eats well. Tuli's friend always offers to listen but says not talking and just being together is fine as well. Those occurrences cause Bel to shrink so that the nasty creature can't manipulate Tuli's efforts for a while.

Humour is also a great way to make your dark topic colourful. Sometimes you find something seemingly absurd during your research and you get one of those "what if" thoughts. Don't be afraid to use that. But to not unintentionally hurt feelings or seem insensitive, you should consult in private a close friend, your expert friend and ideally someone afflicted by your topic. Listen to your gut as well: if a joke doesn't feel right there's probably a reason for that, and you should not use it. After testing in this very private circle, you can test these jokes and separate elements of your game with your target audiences and listen to their opinions as well.

Another way to make your game colourful is to choose a setting that contrasts the dark subject at hand. For DURU, we made the conscious choice to use cute and quirky animal characters and not humans in a realistic world. With our setting we also had the opportunity to create a colourful world that isn't grey and dark like other games about depression which emulate the feeling of this disorder.

Finding metaphors and pictures that convey your message is also a great way to take away the heaviness of your dark topic. Seeing a little dark creature being mean to a cute mole rat is easier to process than seeing said mole rat suffer on its own and closing off.

*Table 1: Step-By-Step-Guide to Creating a Colourful Serious Game*

| **Steps for the Creation of a Colourful Serious Game** | |
|---|---|
| Step 1: Research | Research your topic through web search, books, reports from afflicted people, etc.<br>Find an expert in the field who is willing to share their knowledge and advice for a game.<br>Keep an extra file for colourful, happy or hopeful moments you encounter during your research. |
| Step 2: Define Goals | What is the broader goal of your game?<br>Goals may be: raise awareness, give voice to an inside perspective, explain something complicated in a playful way, give advice, etc. |
| Step 3: Translate Research into Gameplay | Curate your research according to your goal/message. Not everything has to fit into one game!<br>Find mechanics inspired by your research that further an understanding for your topic/help your goal.<br>If that's not possible: create mechanics that convey feelings and emotions related to your topic. |
| Step 4: Make it Colourful | Open your Happy Moment Research File: what fits into your game?<br>What will help take away the weight from your dark/serious topic?<br>Give your game a setting or characters that contrast your dark/serious subject matter.<br>Don't go to extremes if your story and topic can be understood without it. |

## Things to keep in mind

There are some more things to keep in mind that are not related to any specific step. You must keep them in the back of your mind and regularly think of them when looking at your project. As before I will give a summary of them at the end of this part.

During the development of your colourful serious game, you will always go back to your research, and there will always be a need to iterate. When creating any kind of game, testing is a crucial part of the process, but when developing a serious game you pretty much have to test for two things at once. The more general part is testing if the mechanics work and are understood by players: are the controls intuitive, are more tutorials needed, is the art style appealing to the audience? The serious game-specific part is to check if people understand your message and whether your mechanics further this understanding or may be more confusing. I'll give you an example for this from our early-stage testing with DURU.

Originally we designed Bel, our metaphor for depression, as an AI companion that is always there but is not always "bad", as there are in most cases better and worse days when dealing with this disorder. To portray this, on "better days" during the story Bel would actually be helpful as players were able to jump on its back to reach higher platforms. During testing we found that it was confusing our message since the disease is never something helpful. In hindsight it seems obvious, but things are not always that clear during that moment of development, so testing is crucial.

We took this mechanic entirely out of the game. Instead, we put in a shrinking mechanic for Bel: when Tuli is having a good day or another mole rat does something that helps her, Bel would shrink in size. As a tiny creature it was still there, riding along in Tuli's backpack, but it didn't have the power to manipulate Tuli's actions, giving her and players a moment to breathe. Similarly: when another mole rat said or did something that was involuntarily hurtful towards Tuli, Bel would grow and be as nasty as ever. Through testing, we managed to find a clearer way to not only show symptoms but also give players feedback on good and bad behaviour towards someone with depression – one of our main goals!

Another part of our game for which testing was most crucial was the storytelling: the story of our protagonist Tuli is told through animation and picture dialogues/monologues. It took some iterations to find a picture language that was understandable to players. Our first attempt was not that successful, though: players were confused about the many images. Afterwards, we basically built up a dictionary of icons we use, based on common emojis or icons from everyday life. We then used them inside the first part of our game, a kind of tutorial level, and started with very simple "picture phrases" to ease players into the right mind set.

*Figure 3: Examples for "Emoleticons"*

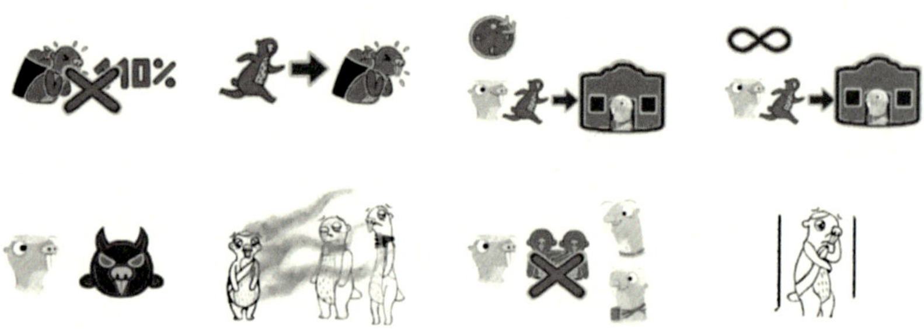


Through continuous work on our picture dictionary, which we called "emoleticons" (because it's mole rats speaking in emoticons), we created a way for players to follow the story while insert their own interpretation and details to make it easier to relate to. Watching "Let's Players" or players at conventions who create dialog from those pictures in their own words is one of my favourite things about DURU.

When asking game developers about testing, especially those with new concepts, they will tell you to do it as early as possible – and that goes double for sensitive subject matter. Start in a circle of friends or with the expert you could hopefully befriend. Even sending along your concept before you had time to establish a first prototype will give you great insight into whether you're on the right track or not.

What goes along with this is double-checking your research and **looking out for misrepresentation**. While it may be true that stereotypes originate from observations in real life, it doesn't mean that there is actual truth to them. Stereotypes originate from an outsider's perception. While you can use them to show exactly that and break them apart, it is crucial to not actually use stereotypes as a basis for a character.

For example: when reading non-scientific articles about depression there is always a picture of a person, mostly in black and white, sitting in a corner, hugging their legs and hiding their face. While it might capture the mood, it is not representative of what a person with depression looks like. Depression can be not being able to decide what kind of bread to buy and leaving the bakery without any. Depression can look like happily chatting with a group of friends while that little dark creature next to you makes you think you are not good enough to be with them. It is that sort of stereotyping that raises expectations of what a person with that disorder looks and acts like, and people being shocked when they hear about their diagnosis. "But they always seem so happy...!" (That is, by the way, a problem everyone with an invisible illness faces. Prominent examples for that might be comedians or actors in comedic roles, like Kurt Krömer or Robin Williams.)

While I will always encourage everybody to try and use **humour** in their **colourful serious game**, I will also advise to be careful about it as well. If your joke contains the topic in some way and is not about something else in your game to lighten the mood, you want it to pass some tests. First one would be your own gut feeling: if you look at your work the next day and there is a weird feeling about it, maybe don't use it. After that you want to show it to your expert friend or another developer who is at least somewhat familiar with the topic. After that maybe discuss it within a community afflicted by that topic. As with all things: a single voice, even from a person who is afflicted by your topic, does not present that whole group of people. On the other hand: even with these measures you can't be certain that no person will be offended.

So... what now? Well, you can make sure to communicate that your story and the joke within it is just one story, one perspective on that topic. In case of humorous works about depression, there are some German authors that were confronted with questions of whether it should be allowed to laugh about depression in their books. To which they answered: "Of course!" One example for that is Tobias Katze, a German author who wrote the book "Morgen ist leider auch noch ein Tag" which translates to "Unfortunately, tomorrow is another day".

The thing to be mindful about here is that nobody is laughing about the topic of depression or the illness itself, but rather about the weird situations that can occur when dealing with it. For quite a few people, including these authors, it was their way of dealing with all the terribleness that came with their illness: finding the humour in a dark situation. In that way you can use it for your colourful serious game as well. Just make sure your joke is not aimed at the topic itself but rather at a specific, weird situation that comes from it.

*Table 2: Colorful Serious Games Checklist*

| **Checklist** | |
|---|---|
| Test & Adjust | As early as possible, test your prototype. While watching others play, ask yourself these questions:<br>Do players know which subjects your game is about without you telling them?<br>Are your mechanics clear regarding your topic or do they confuse it or your message? |
| Be careful with clichés & stereotypes | Keep an eye out for misrepresentation. If something is portrayed a certain way, often it does not necessarily mean that it is representative of that topic/person. Keep in mind that stereotypes always originate from an outsider's perception |
| Double check your jokes | Humour is a great way to connect your players to your topic and/or characters. When using jokes, be mindful what they are aimed at and how they are perceived. As a first thing, make sure they are not making fun of the topic itself but rather, e.g. a weird situation that occurs |

## The potential of colorful serious games

After reaching a point where I could talk quite openly about my depression, I found that many people were curious about it. I joke that my introduction at dates was "Hi, I'm Kerstin. I have depression, so when I don't respond to a text for a long time it's because of that, not because of you". And after putting that out there in such a blatant way, we would have a laugh and an interesting conversation about misconceptions of depression and mental health in general, not just mine but the other person's as well. Humour and a certain light-heartedness are great ice breakers, not only in conversations but also in movies or games about dark or serious topics. You immediately create a safe space for people not to feel judged about their own problems and guide them into an open-minded space.

When dealing with topics of that nature, it is hard to find the intrinsic motivation to educate oneself about it. We've all got only so many hours in a day, and for some it takes quite some willpower to use them to learn about something that carries a sense of unpleasantness. In education there is the concept of "stealth learning" (Sharp, 2012). It describes a situation in which an untraditional tool or a game is used to teach something to students without them realizing they are learning. The same principle can, of course, be applied to games that are commercial in nature and not specifically intended for use in a classroom or a young audience.

Games are an amazing medium to present a topic, whether serious or not, and create an easy access to approach it. And when you choose to make it a colourful experience on top of that, chances are you reach more people; even those who were not aware of that topic to begin with.

## The lessons learned

DURU was our first colourful serious game, with which we learned some lessons that we'd like to share. They are more about communication about your game and not the game development process itself.

When we first started pitching DURU and saying it is a game about depression, people had the expectation of it being a therapy game. We never said it targets people with depression, but saying "game" and "depression" in a sentence already put an image into most people's mind. We learned that when it comes to a game like this, it is as important to communicate **what your game is** as well **as what it is not**. This goes especially for games about mental disorders, but I can see this problem also occur with other topics. Depending on your game it might be a good idea to communicate your goals right at the start of your pitch and only after that move on to talking about the game itself before an image can form in the heads of your audience.

The full title of our game is DURU – ABOUT MOLE RATS AND DEPRESSION. This was more of an accidental choice, but we went with it after receiving good feedback at exhibitions and conventions. People read it while passing our booth. Then they stopped and came back because they wanted to double-check the title and became very curious: depression and our colourful art style at first glance shouldn't go well together. We also had very open conversations with people feeling safe to talk about their experience with this illness and were glad that this "wasn't another greyscale game" about that topic. But what worked so well in the open wild of reality didn't translate well into the digital world. Here we found that people who never heard about our game were scared off by that heavy word. For our next game we decided to go more with the stealth learning approach and hide our true goal when it comes to marketing the finished product to consumers.

When it came to our Kickstarter campaign, on the other hand, we found that being open about our goal attracted a lot of people outside of the gaming world. We had quite a few people new to Kickstarter who supported with us. And we had people like this one lady who wrote us a message that "she doesn't know how to play games but thinks that it is a great way for younger people to learn about depression". When you plan on making a crowdfunding campaign or explore other routes of securing funding, you'll certainly reach a wider audience when you are open about your topic and your goal.

The most important and rather beautiful lesson we learned is that we want to continue to make this kind of game. It is not only fulfilling as a developer to provide both entertainment and education at the same time: you will also make a lot of connections with people and provide them a safe space to talk about that topic which is so important to them or that is maybe affecting their life directly. You might also reach that one person who wasn't interested in games but will pick up yours because it is about something they can relate to. And as a game developer, what can be more fulfilling than this.

## References

Buday, J., Neumann, M., Heidingerová, J., Michalec, J., Podgorná, G., Mareš, T., Pol, M., Mahrík, J., Vranková, S., Kališová, L., Anders, M. (2022). Depiction of mental illness and psychiatry in popular video games over the last 20 years. *Frontiers in Psychiatryk,* 13. https://doi.org/10.3389/fpsyt.2022.967992

Hazel, J. (2019). How to Represent Mental Illness in Games, *Game Developer Conference 2019*, https://www.gdcvault.com/play/1026319/How-to-Represent-Mental-Illness

Sharp, L. A. (2012). Stealth Learning: Unexpected Learning Opportunities through Games. *Journal of Instructional Research*, 1, https://files.eric.ed.gov/fulltext/EJ1127609.pdf

World Health Organisation (2023). *Depressive disorder (depression)*. https://www.who.int/news-room/fact-sheets/detail/depression

# Something Beautiful is Going to Happen

## Disco Elysium and the Depiction of Mental Health Struggles in Gaming

*Samantha Accettulli*

Although video games have been tackling topics related to psychology for several decades now, it can be difficult to integrate these themes into a game in a way that would attract players who do not necessarily have an interest in exploring them. Disco Elysium (ZA/UM, 2019), a game that is initially presented as a detective story but that is much more than that, is an example of how this integration can occur successfully. Numerous players have written about their unique experiences with the game, even in comparison to other games that address similar themes—including learning more about the workings of their own brains, the benefits of psychotherapy and of feeling heard and understood when struggling with depression, substance abuse, and suicidality (Corrigan, 2020; Diggins, 2021; Kuhn, 2022; Magestro, 2021; Walker, 2021). What is it about this murder mystery game that is leading people to have these revelations? Exploring some of its unique development elements, aspects of its structure, and philosophies that influence Disco Elysium may provide guidance for developers looking to make games that are heavily mental health-informed without explicitly being about exploring mental health struggles.

### What is *Disco Elysium*?

Disco Elysium is an isometric role-playing game developed and published by ZA/UM and released on multiple platforms in 2019, with a major update that occurred in 2021 that added voice acting and additional questlines. In Disco Elysium players control an initially unnamed protagonist who wakes up in his underwear in a hostel room with almost complete amnesia. Through discussions in the game and the discovery of certain objects, we come to find out that he is Harry Du Bois, a detective in the Revachol Citizens Militia, and he has been sent to figure out who killed a man who is currently hanging from a tree behind the hostel. We also find out that Harry struggles with alcohol and other substances, and that he may have been attempting to kill himself prior to the beginning of the game. The area of Martinaise, a district of the city of Revachol that the game takes place in, is in the middle of a bloody conflict between a large corporation and the local union. With his partner Kim Kitsuragi, who has never met the detective before, Harry strives to solve the murder, figure out who he is, and what happened to make him lose his memory, while attempting to prevent the tensions in the area from boiling over into outright warfare.

In order to solve these mysteries, the player of Disco Elysium spends their time investigating areas and talking to non-player characters. The game is deeply text-based, to such a degree that some consider it to resemble a playable novel more than a video game. Unlike in most other role-playing games, our beleaguered detective is not a professional combatant —there is effectively no playable combat in the game at all. In lieu of defeating enemies in battle, the game equips Harry with numerous mental tools.

## Skills, Thought Cabinet, Political System, Copotypes

*Figure 1: Skills Menu in DISCO ELYSIUM*

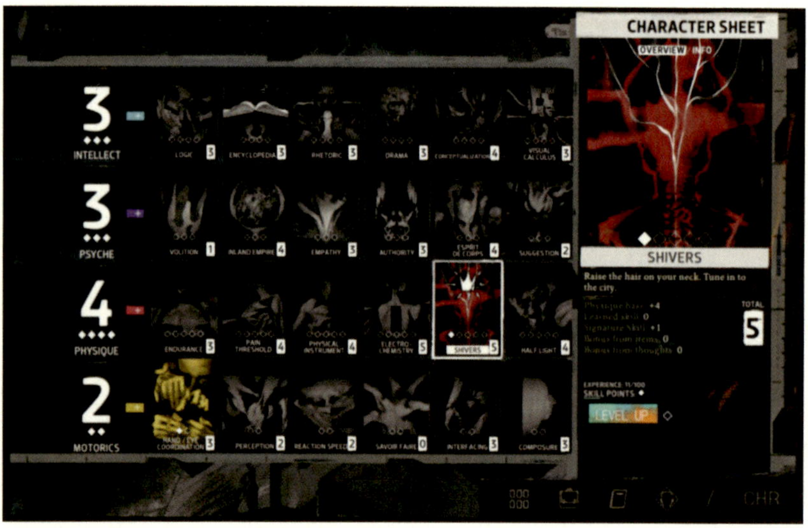


Screenshot by author

In DISCO ELYSIUM, much of the interaction occurs between Harry's skills, which replace the more traditional RPG character sheet with different stat points (fig. 1). While the skills act as representations of the strengths or weaknesses of some of

Harry's abilities, they also all function as aspects of his personality. They range from more recognizable qualities like Endurance and Empathy to more esoteric ones like Inland Empire—an aspect that allows Harry to connect with elements of the world that may seem paranormal. All of them are illustrated and voiced as independent characters and, depending on the amount of points each skill is allotted, they might choose to comment on a particular situation or stay silent. (Figs. 2 and 3) Additionally, the skills have to pass checks from time to time, as in a traditional RPG. Passing and failing these checks can lead to highly entertaining results.

*Figure 2 + 3: The "Empathy" Skill*

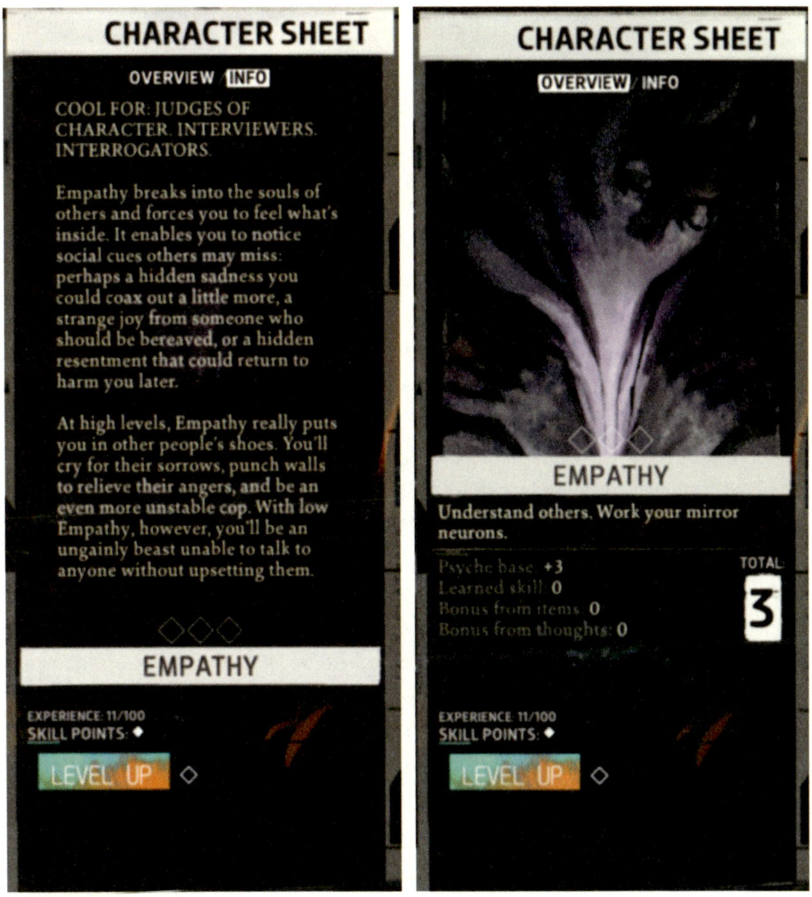
CHARACTER SHEET
OVERVIEW / INFO
COOL FOR: JUDGES OF CHARACTER. INTERVIEWERS. INTERROGATORS.
Empathy breaks into the souls of others and forces you to feel what's inside. It enables you to notice social cues others may miss: perhaps a hidden sadness you could coax out a little more, a strange joy from someone who should be bereaved, or a hidden resentment that could return to harm you later.
At high levels, Empathy really puts you in other people's shoes. You'll cry for their sorrows, punch walls to relieve their angers, and be an even more unstable cop. With low Empathy, however, you'll be an ungainly beast unable to talk to anyone without upsetting them.
EMPATHY
EXPERIENCE: 11/100
SKILL POINTS:
LEVEL UP
CHARACTER SHEET
OVERVIEW / INFO
EMPATHY
Understand others. Work your mirror neurons.
Psyche base: +3
Learned skill: 0
Bonus from items: 0
Bonus from thoughts: 0
TOTAL
3
EXPERIENCE: 11/100
SKILL POINTS:
LEVEL UP

Screenshots by author

Sometimes, the skills directly disagree with each other and cause Harry to doubt some of them, as in a portion of the game that involves him interrogating a clever and beautiful woman who does not want Harry to know too much about her:

> VOLITION – I have bad news for you.
> YOU – What?
> VOLITION – You know these guys?
> LOGIC – Who, me?
> DRAMA – Yes, you. He's talking about you, you boring stiff.
> VOLITION – You too.
> DRAMA – Me? What did I do? I'm merely a master thespian...
> VOLITION – These guys are compromised. She's got them singing along to her tune. The little bleeps and bloops you trust for info – you can't trust them anymore. (ZA/UM, 2021).

Some players have associated the skill system—and the way the skills talk amongst themselves and to Harry—with various mental health concepts, including Internal Family Systems (IFS) and its related parts language (Rijnders, 2023), living as a system as might be seen in Dissociative Identity Disorder (DID) and Other Specified Dissociative Disorder (OSDD; Go, 2022), and hearing voices and experiencing delusions (Delüzyon_Emekçisi, 2024). The division of Harry's psyche into multiple aspects in the form of the Skills has been relatable to these players, whether this is due to the normal human experience of feeling like multiple parts (as seen in IFS) or experiences that do not align with a typical sense of self, such as distinct identities (as experienced in DID or OSDD), or experiences of psychosis. The popularity of a playthrough by the therapist and streamer Euro Brady may indicate a desire of the playerbase to dig deeper into these mental health themes, with the most popular upload of his analysis receiving over 350,000 views (Euro Brady, n.d.).

The Thought Cabinet takes the place of a typical RPG skill modification menu and allows players to gain more understanding of the world of Elysium and Harry's past (Fig. 4). During the design process, the game's lead writer Robert Kurvitz wanted to come up with a way to represent the more traditional RPG experience of killing an enemy and harvesting their items in a way that reflects the conversation-heavy style of the game. He asked himself: "What is the loot of conversations?...The answer is ideas" (GameSpot, 2020). When a thought is "internalized" in the cabinet, it generally provides some kind of modification to Harry's in-game stats, similar to equipping a weapon or piece of armor in another game. While these thoughts can change aspects of how likely Harry is to succeed or fail at various experiences in-game, they also often contain information about Harry's past or the world in which he exists. Each thought is labeled as a "problem" when it is initially identified. After a thought has been processed and internalized, Harry arrives at a solution and the corresponding bonuses or penalties are applied. There are a limited number of slots in which to keep internalized thoughts, so players must be selective about which ones they will keep or discard. In this way, players are encouraged to see how choosing to focus one's mind on certain aspects of itself or of the world influences one's worldview. Many of the thoughts also have very introspective writing that mirrors a novel much more than it resembles a traditional video game.

*Figure 4: The "Thought Cabinet" Menu*

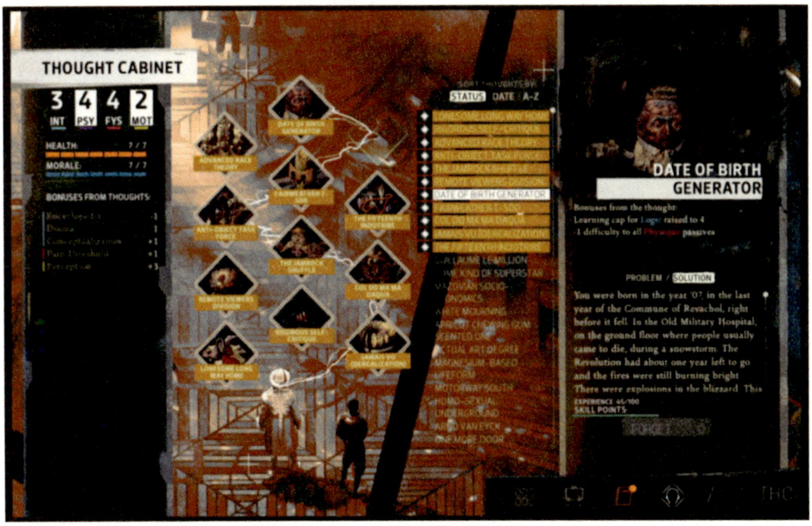
THOUGHT CABINET
3 4 4 2
INT PSY FYS MOT
HEALTH
MORALE
BONUSES FROM THOUGHTS
STATUS DATE A-Z
DATE OF BIRTH GENERATOR
PROBLEM / SOLUTION
You were born in the year '07, in the last year of the Commune of Revachol, right before it fell. In the Old Military Hospital, on the ground floor where people usually came to die, during a snowstorm. The Revolution had about one year left to go and the fires were still burning bright. There were explosions in the blizzard. This
SKILL POINTS

Screenshot by author

For instance, the thought "Finger on the Eject Button" can only occur if Harry has talked to a pair of young twins whose father appears to have died by suicide and validating that suicide is something that makes sense to him, stating to the twins: "It's okay to kill yourself, you know. I'm gonna blow my brains out. Gonna close this one final case and then *blam* – I'm outta here." If the player chooses to begin internalizing this thought, they are provided with a somewhat hopeful paragraph about contemplating how much other people might miss Harry if he were to die. From this internalization, Harry receives a boost to his Authority and Suggestion skills, indicating that he becomes stronger when thinking about killing himself. After the thought is internalized, the "solution" that Harry comes up with is that suicide might be the best option for him, all stat bonuses are removed, and the player is offered the choice to die by suicide every night as Harry goes to sleep until the game ends or the thought is "forgotten" and removed from the Cabinet. This does not influence the larger story, the gameplay, or Harry's journey, but speaks to the idea that Harry's suicidality might be a part of him for the rest of his life regardless of his success or failure at solving the case—an idea that could ring true for the myriad of people who struggle with chronic suicidal ideation.

Disco Elysium also features a system for determining Harry's political affiliation, something that is heavily woven into the game, as multiple political systems are represented by various characters' interests and motivations. Harry is offered dialogue options related to the ideologies of communism, fascism, moralism, or ultraliberalism. Each of these alignments has their own special quest in the Final Cut edition of the game and, once one has been completed, all others become off-limits for the rest of that particular playthrough. The function of judging the player's playstyle without making it explicit is somewhat unusual considering that games are commonly expected to explain their mechanics clearly. In a post on the development blog about the creation of the political system, the ZA/UM community manager made it clear that this subtle judgment is by design, stating that

> "Disco Elysium is, in many ways, a personality test. There are always little integers in the background, counting everything you say" (Woodford, 2019).

This aspect of the game provides a window into the potential of receiving information about yourself as a player without the awareness of being "tested".

This is also related to the various "copotypes" in the game, which are descriptors for Harry's personality traits—i.e. what type of cop he is. The player can choose to emphasize one over the others in their responses. These manifest as labels like "Superstar Cop", a version of Harry who sees himself in an extremely positive light, or "Boring Cop", which involves almost always picking the most lawful option, even in ambiguous circumstances. These can also function as commentary on playstyle. For example, a player who apologizes frequently in the game will be given the mantle of "Sorry Cop", which can lead to an in-game thought that lists numerous unpleasant actions Harry has committed over the course of his life and the opportunities to improve that he has squandered. The description states that "You let misery win. And it will keep on winning till you die – or overcome it". The player's attempt to make Harry a better person by apologizing is effectively rendered empty unless he (or rather, the player) changes his actions. The variety of options available pushes far beyond the typical selection system in many RPGs that can sometimes break down into a good response/neutral response/evil response dynamic.

## How can video games be used to interface with mental health? The case of *Hellblade*

Hellblade: Senua's Sacrifice (Ninja Theory, 2017) received accolades for its well-informed portrayal of psychosis.

In a study using HELLBLADE, researchers showed how the game can help reduce the stigma of mental health issues and increase empathy towards those suffering from them (Ferchaud et al., 2020). The study produced numerous significant results, including data that supports the idea that people may benefit more from these effects when they are actually playing a game rather than simply watching a playthrough. Their work supports the idea that there is something unique about engaging in media from a monadic lens, in which there is little separation between the player and the character they are engaging with, rather than a dyadic lens, where the person engaging with the character always has some level of distance—as in books, movies, and television shows. In short, a monadic lens can increase a media consumer's identification with a character (Ferchaud et al., 2020). While DISCO ELYSIUM presents occasional fourth-wall breaking comments, the dialogue does not reference the idea of separation between the player and Harry, simply referring to his inner core as "You".

Increased identification with a character who is struggling with mental health issues was shown to promote lower levels of desire for social distance from people who are dealing with mental health struggles, and being able to take the perspective of another person or character promotes a larger sense of social acceptance of stigmatized groups (Ferchaud et al., 2020). This seems to produce an increased sense of empathy towards both the self and others, especially as increased identification with a game character can temporarily reduce a person's sense of their own-self concept, which may allow new ways of viewing the self and others to enter their mind. Because this happens unconsciously as a person is engaging with a video game character, there is some evidence supporting the idea that video games that are not explicitly designed as mental health interventions may be useful for delivering anti-stigma messages, as this may bypass negative reactions that could result from a person feeling like a moral or message is being delivered to them (Ferchaud et al., 2020).

## What facets of *Disco Elysium*'s development make it unique?

While DISCO ELYSIUM is situated within a much larger universe that its creators had already mapped out years prior to ever considering creating a video game, there are some qualities that are unique to the game itself, which may explain the deep connections that some players have experienced. Today, ZA/UM is a game development studio that has undergone significant personnel changeover since the creation of

Disco Elysium. However, ZA/UM existed previously as the name of an artists' collective that wanted to create a new cultural movement. The collective also engaged in extensive tabletop roleplaying in a universe of their own creation that would later serve as the setting for the game. Many of the game's writers and developers were original members of this collective (Izual, 2019). Kurvitz stated that, "I want people to expect a lot more from video game writing... I want there to be fictional universes that talk about our own real life experiences. About the political problems we're facing, the geopolitical structures around us, the problems of the modern world, etc... Universes which actually equip us with life tools and provide context for what's happening to us" (Izual, 2019).

While there are multiple writers credited with working on Disco Elysium and the game's creation involved consultation with a researcher specifically focusing on subjects like psychology and forensics, Kurvitz and his collaborators have spoken about some of the ways that his difficulties with his own mental health informed the creation of Harry Du Bois (Morton, 2019).

Kurvitz, of Estonian origin, published the first commercially available work in Disco Elysium's universe, the novel titled Püha ja õudne lõhn in the original language (often translated as Sacred and Terrible Air) in 2013. After the book only sold about a thousand copies, he found himself struggling with alcohol abuse and having difficulties engaging in creative pursuits. After one of Disco Elysium's other creators, Kaur Kender, suggested that he turn the world he was creating into a video game, Kurvitz got his substance use issues into a more manageable place and was able to eventually publish the game despite never having made one before. While much of the world and lore of Elysium was already created by ZA/UM, many of Harry's specific experiences seem to parallel one of his creators' lives, which lends his struggles a kind of realism that other games that aim to tackle mental health topics from a more clinical lens may not as accurately depict.

Additionally, the game is heavily inspired by its creators' experiences of growing up in the 1990s in post-Soviet Estonia, a time that they characterize as "gruesome" but giving rise to interesting art that was attempting to reckon with the new world Estonians were living in (Wiltshire, 2020). Disco Elysium is grounded in a very real-feeling environment by avoiding typical fantasy or sci-fi world templates, and instead mixing old and new technology, squalor and splendor, and focusing on the struggle of unions as capitalists attempt to take power from laborers. An Iraqi player stated that the game captured the feeling of growing up in his war-torn home country better than anything he had ever seen, stating that "There's so much attention and thus so much love everywhere in this game for humans and what humans do. Doesn't matter if they might all get shot, blown up, or wiped clean by pale in a couple years. Doesn't matter if they brought it all on themselves. Right here, in this moment, they are human, and so they matter" (Beamoon2016, 2023).

## What have *Disco Elysium* players said about their experiences?

Numerous authors have written about the ways that DISCO ELYSIUM gave them a new perspective on their own mental health or on the experience of dealing with mental health struggles generally. There are a large number of anecdotes and personal experiences that players have written about in a variety of spaces, including on blogs, social media, Steam reviews, and even journal articles, with some segments of particularly thoughtful blog posts included in this chapter. One author described feeling aspects of themselves reflected in Harry. By viewing him as a deeply flawed individual who is at times volatile and harms other people, while still being worthy of care and accomplishments that are meaningful to him and to others, playing DISCO ELYSIUM made them feel more convinced that going to therapy could be worth it for them (Corrigan, 2020). Another player described how the game represents the struggle of talking about one's mental health difficulties while acknowledging the impact it may have on others. In an essay about their experience with the game, they reflected on the moment in which Harry (and therefore the player) has the choice to respond to encouragement from Kim by saying "I don't want to get better, I want to get worse". The author noted that they did not want to select this option because of how it would make Kim feel and how strongly their internal experience of trying to select the "right" dialogue option mirrored their own experience of hiding how hopeless they really felt when dealing with depression themselves so as to not negatively affect others (Diggins, 2021). Another player wrote about how Harry's desires to self-destruct and his memory loss mirrored some of their own experience with depression, often having the sense that they have struggled to establish an identity that is not based in being useful to others or fulfilling the objectives they feel have been placed on them (Magestro, 2021).

Others have written about how the game's structure influenced their playstyle in ways that made it feel much more difficult to act in ways that were not personally aligned with who they are due to the guilt arising from causing harm to Harry or other characters. Some have spoken of the difficulty of conducting a playthrough of the game that involves selecting cruel or chaotic options, as their own personal feelings towards hurting Kim or other characters were so unpleasant that they have not been able to fully engage in a "bad" playthrough (Kuhn, 2022). Another player wrote about their experience with the game measuring the character's mental health not in terms of "sanity" or other meter systems sometimes used in games but in terms of morale, leading to Harry's psychological "death" if he becomes too despondent or loses belief in himself (Walker, 2021). While they had personally found it enjoyable at times to push Harry and see how outlandish some of his responses could get in the game even as they damaged him, the author also named how connected they felt to the idea that things in their life could be going well when it came to outside markers, but that lacking belief in themselves could still damage their ability to function.

Research has also been conducted to attempt to qualify exactly what players are responding to in Disco Elysium. In Klimczyk (2021), study participants who had played Disco Elysium completed a questionnaire in order to identify ways in which a player's completion of the game might influence their life story narrative. The narratives players provided were interpreted via hermeneutic analysis and phenomenological analysis in order to identify significant themes that continued to influence their lives and views of themselves and contexts in which some of these themes arose. One study participant viewed themselves as a therapist to Harry, attempting to pick choices that were most likely to lead to positive outcomes for him and desiring to help him achieve more stability even as the player remained separate from Harry rather than feeling similarity in their identities. Another participant viewed Harry as initially frightening and suspicious because he lived such a different life from her and dealt with problems she had not personally experienced (such as substance use). As she spent more time in his world, however, she developed an increased sense of empathy for the character and more compassion towards herself for her own mental health struggles. While both players retained a sense of separation from Harry, both experienced an increase in their understanding of the perspective of a person dealing with some of his issues and named a desire to try to save him from his suffering even if they initially viewed him negatively.

## A game grounded in powerlessness

Many Disco Elysium players who start the game expecting a typical experience of saving the world and experiencing a generally positive ending may be shocked by the journey they end up taking.

The murderer is revealed to be a character that is heavily related to the political themes of the game, not someone that the player could have reasonably guessed prior to the very end of the story. The central mystery of the game thus breaks one of the classic rules of detective fiction, which is that the criminal must be a character involved in the early part of a story (Knox, 1929). Many of the larger conflicts between the union and the corporation and other actors in the world are not solvable in-game. There are inescapable encounters and characters who will die regardless of how the player handles the situation. There is no way for Harry to win his ex-fiancée back. Attempts to contact her end up damaging him and evoking feelings of frustration and sadness in her. This is exemplified by a thought from Harry's skill Shivers. This skill allows him to hear a voice stated to be the personification of Revachol itself and to sometimes witness or hear experiences that occurred in the past or will occur in the future. Through this particular thought, Harry finds out that the city is going to be destroyed by a nuclear bomb in a few decades and that a mysterious fog called The Pale is spreading over the world that will literally consume it all a few years after the explosion. Many of these factors could lead to the game being viewed as bleak, depressing, or hopeless, especially as many games are grounded in the inherent special qualities of their protagonists and their ability to turn the tide of massive events.

Disco Elysium also keeps the health and influence of larger systems in mind as it depicts the struggles of Harry and others to get by in the world. If he is unable to find enough money to get a hostel room during the first night of the game, he will die in the cold. Numerous characters are subject to economic factors that keep them separated from loved ones, harm their ability to pursue things that are important to them, or leave them living in rundown buildings or dependent on rich benefactors. While Harry can positively influence the life of Cuno, a young boy dealing with an abusive father, substance use issues, and poverty, he is unable to meaningfully change his future other than potentially securing him a position in the Revachol Citizens' Militia, which may just be replacing one defective system with another. Racism, sexism, homophobia, xenophobia, and other harmful systems of thought show up frequently in the game, sometimes in very obvious ways (there is a character named Racist Lorry Driver) and sometimes in ways that can feel both realistic and heartbreaking (like getting to know Lena, a kind older woman who turns out to believe unpleasant theories about race). Even when the player selects dialogue options that challenge other characters' biases or allows them to defend Kim, who is biracial and sometimes the target of these racist remarks, it is still possible to fail a check and automatically call him a racial slur, revealing that having grown up in a racist environment may always influence Harry. By centering the complexity of trying to improve as a person while the systems around you struggle to function, the game keeps Harry's difficulties grounded in a reality that may feel very familiar to players.

## Tackling complex themes in unique ways

In addition to probing aspects of mental health such as depression or existential dread, Disco Elysium very specifically leans into aspects of the character's experience that can be complicated to depict in any type of media, let alone one like gaming that has to account for many choices a player could make. Some of the more specific psychological themes that emerge when playing the game include substance use, the intersection between personal experience and political ideology, and trauma and recovery.

## Substance use

The depiction of Harry's struggles with addiction differs quite a bit from other games that attempt to render its effects in an in-game way. A more common representation of addiction is featured in the game LISA: THE PAINFUL (Dingaling Productions, 2014), which includes characters who are addicted to a substance called Joy and experience significant changes to their in-game stats when in withdrawal, which is reliably relieved by taking more Joy. In DISCO ELYSIUM, however, there is no significant downside to abstaining from substance use. Some of Harry's stats are certainly enhanced by smoking, drinking, or taking pills, but it is really up to the player to decide if Harry will enjoy the bonuses that come from using the substances or attempt to pass checks on their own.

The main way in which addiction is depicted is in the form of the voices of the Skills as well as Harry's Horrific Necktie, an item of clothing that can speak to him if some of his stats are high enough. Harry can experience numerous intrusive thoughts related to substances, including seeing alcohol that has poured onto a table and wanting to lick it up, the Electrochemistry skill frequently chiming in to let him know that a substance is in the room with him, and his Necktie encouraging him to party and connect back to his old disco days. By allowing Harry to continue functioning in-game without substances and depicting much of the internal battle of whether or not to use as a mental one, the game offers a more grounded picture of what it is like to struggle with substance use rather than one that operates on life or death stakes.

While players are free to either use the various substances in the game to improve Harry's performance or to abstain from them in the service of setting Harry down a path of sobriety without much judgment in the game either way, there is a thought in the Thought Cabinet that can feel quite impactful. If the player does agree with a particular in-game option of wanting to get sober and internalizes the "Waste Land of Reality" thought, they are provided with a message that states "Congrats – you're sober...Full recovery will take years, though. It'll be depressing. And it'll be boring. Don't expect any further rewards or handclaps. This is how normal people are all the time." By offering a realistic look at many people's experiences of sobriety, which can be heavily characterized by a sense of increased boredom and a lack of recognition of the struggle and drudgery that can accompany having to deliberately choose abstinence from substances forever, the game challenges more romanticized depictions of overcoming addiction. Additionally, by still making it possible to achieve a positive ending in the game even if the player does choose to use substances, it makes players consider that Harry can still be a person worthy of growth and new experiences even if he does not recover.

## Political ideology

While DISCO ELYSIUM was created by a development team significantly influenced by communism, with writer Helen Hindpere specifically thanking Karl Marx and Friedrich Engels for their "political education" during ZA/UM's acceptance speech at The Game Awards (Jackson, 2019), it depicts all four of its political alignments with deep insight and heavy connections to the psychology of the specific version of Harry who might find himself drawn most heavily in one of the four directions. Communism is depicted as an ideology that both inspired a violent revolution but also has the power to create hope and transformation, even though the game posits that any progress will be laughably slow. Fascism is depicted as heavily tying in with feelings of rejection by women, racism, and a desire for things to return to the "good old days", but the game is still able to depict these unpleasant topics with nuance and to show how someone who feels hurt by the world could be led down that particular path. Moralism, an ideology heavily based in centrism and incrementalism, might be the alignment that a person trying to play apolitically ends up with, but the thought that accompanies it effectively states that a centrist believes in nothing. Ultraliberalism is tied in with the pursuit of wealth and does give Harry access to slightly more money but is also looked down upon by almost every other character he can encounter.

By depicting these political alignments as potential belief systems that could all spring forth from the same person, DISCO ELYSIUM is able to demonstrate the way that experience can predispose someone to align more heavily with one particular philosophy than others, but that each person ultimately has to make the choice to fully commit. Various dialogue options in the game provide points in each of the political alignments, but players may be unsure of which alignment the choice aligns with until after they have made it. The ability of the player to stumble into Harry's politics without entirely realizing it can likely increase empathy for people ending up in any of the particular camps even when the game explicitly does not approve of some of these ideologies.

## Trauma and recovery

In addition to some of the aforementioned ways that collective trauma is represented in the game in the form of sociopolitical and economic strife, DISCO ELYSIUM is very specific about the ways that painful experiences throughout a person's life can predispose them to experience the world in unpleasant ways. Harry exists as a character who is capable of harm to others and who has been deeply harmed by others and his circumstances. Through the Thought Cabinet and the reflections of characters who know him, we find out that Harry likely lost his parents early in life, that all of his childhood friends have passed away, that he felt so insecure in his relationship with his ex-fiancée Dora Ingerlund that he completely shifted careers, and that he has lost his memory in similar ways before, which is potentially related to his substance use. All of these experiences add up to how he presents in the game as the player encounters him, existing with a mind that is very attuned to the beauty of the world and intensely curious, but also suspicious of others and deeply afraid of being hurt.

Even if the player makes choices for Harry that are attempting to make him a better person, we find out that he has engaged in numerous actions that have led to physical and emotional damage to others. Some have occurred in the context of his role as a police officer and would even be considered police brutality, such as severely physically harming a suspect. Others have occurred in the context of his personal life, as the player discovers if they attempt to reach out to Dora via a phone call and are greeted with a kind of sadness and resignation from her that makes it clear that Harry has reached out before and she does not want to hear from him. The player is also able to interact with Harry's ex-partner Jean Vicquemare at various points in the game, who displays a willingness to defend Harry from certain consequences even as he gives him a verbal lashing at times and indicates how badly he feels he has been hurt by Harry's actions.

Under the best of circumstances, DISCO ELYSIUM takes a realistic yet optimistic approach to the healing of Harry's trauma. Characters make reference to the idea that mental health services in Revachol are underdeveloped, so Harry is unlikely to receive actual mental health care as he recovers. He is unable to create the conditions to get back into a relationship with Dora, even as memories of her haunt him throughout the game. Jean's view of Harry can become more positive by the end of the game, but there is no impression that Harry will be instantly forgiven for everything that has happened. While it is impossible to undo his actions or go back to the way his life was before, Harry is able to engage in post-traumatic growth, the positive psychological changes that can occur in the aftermath of a significant event that can lead to increased self-awareness, a more open attitude towards others, and a greater appreciation of life (Dell'Osso et al, 2022).

Game scholar Thomas Spies (2021) has interpreted Harry's story as a representation of Camus' view of absurdism, in that he is offered three choices for how to cope with the mess that his life has become: kill himself, have a kind of blind hope that relies on things that may not come to pass, or accept the inherent absurdity of life and make choices within what is available to him. While some portions of the game may end up feeling more like damage control for players rather than a true victory, Harry is still able to make significant differences in the lives of people that he intersects with or even just in his own concept of the world. He is able to deliver the news to a woman that her missing husband has passed away rather than leaving her wondering forever. He is able to engage in artistic expression by painting a mural on a wall that permanently remains. He is able to help some local ravers start a dance club in an abandoned church, a task that has induced joyful feelings in many players when they are finally able to see Harry and Kim dancing and celebrating even in the midst of tragedy. And he is able to meet the Insulindian Phasmid, a cryptid whose existence is hotly debated throughout the course of the game but ends up being tied into a larger sense of Harry's attempts to try to find meaning. Only through this encounter is he able to deliver the line "I'm glad to be me – an incredibly sensitive instrument", a statement closer to self-actualization than anything else in the game.

## What can developers learn about incorporating psychological themes into their games from *Disco Elysium*?

There are numerous factors unique to DISCO ELYSIUM that would be difficult to replicate in other games. Even so, referring to a game as "Disco-like" has become a selling point for games such as CITIZEN SLEEPER (Jump Over the Age, 2022), NORCO (Geography of Robots, 2022), PENTIMENT (Obsidian Entertainment, 2022), and other role-playing games and visual novels released in its wake that deemphasize or completely eliminate combat and have a focus on complex characters and themes (Colp, 2022).

However, there are some ideas emphasized in this exploration that may be useful in the creation of games with a heavy psychological influence:

1. The game systems are also the means by which the player is encouraged to learn more about Harry's psychology. By taking known RPG tropes like character sheets and abilities and giving them a unique perspective, players obtain information about the organization of Harry's mind without explicit encouragement.
2. It is important to have diverse creators involved in the creation of games and incorporating unique and new perspectives can lead to extremely positive results. DISCO ELYSIUM would be a very different game had it not had the same specific cultural and personal influences, and identifying what unique life experiences game developers can bring to the table can be pivotal for creating new works.
3. While it is very helpful to have games created to explicitly address mental health topics such as the reduction of stigma and the generation of new tools for reaching people who are working to improve their mental health, it may be equally helpful to examine how these topics can be woven in to games that are not "about" mental health. By bringing players in through one door and then leading them out through a completely different one, it may be possible to get a wider audience thinking about psychological topics than people who might pick up a game "about depression".

4. While more and more games have sought to incorporate mature themes, Disco Elysium is a reminder that developers need not shy away from addressing heavy and complicated topics, and that an interactive story may have unique potential to give players new perspectives when it comes to multifaceted situations. While it is not a game for all audiences, the way that it has already begun to inspire the creation of other similar titles and entire journal issues devoted to exploring its themes may offer some proof of its influence (Apperley, T., & Ozimek, A., 2021).
5. Providing opportunities for players to learn more about themselves through playing a game could be a way that video games end up directly interfacing with the goal of improving the mental health of their players. While some might be offended by a game calling them a fascist or poking fun at their shallow understanding of feminism, the potential for a player to learn something new about themselves without being aware that they are being assessed opens up huge potential for unbiased self-reflection.

Disco Elysium is a game so large and complex that writing about it could likely fill its own book. By taking lessons from the boldness of its creators and the empathy and understanding that is heavily baked into the game, however, anyone who chooses to play it may be able to learn things about how they can create art with more nuance that truly engages with the world it is made in rather than only providing an escapist fantasy.

## References

Apperley, T., & Ozimek, A. (Eds.) (2021). Disco Elysium: Special issue on Baltic Screen Media Review. Baltic Screen Media Review, 9. https://sciendo.com/issue/BSMR/9/1

[Beamoon2016]. (2023, July 24). Never thought I'd read a story that so effectively captures why life in a broken system is worth living [Online forum post]. Retrieved from https://www.reddit.com/r/DiscoElysium/comments/158jbx1/never_thought_id_read_a_story_that_so_effectively/

Colp, T. (2022, December 29). The fate of Disco Elysium 2 is uncertain, but these games make up for it. PC Gamer. https://www.pcgamer.com/disco-elysiums-influence-on-games-grows-despite-its-sequels-uncertain-fate/

Corrigan, H. (2020, January 14). Disco Elysium taught me I need therapy. SUPERJUMP. https://medium.com/super-jump/disco-elysium-taught-me-i-need-therapy-1f5c9b09ce6b

Dell'Osso, L., Lorenzi, P., Nardi, B., Carmassi, C., Carpita, B., (2022). Post traumatic growth (PTG) in the frame of traumatic experiences. *Clinical Neuropsychiatry*, 19(6), 390- 393.

Delüzyon_Emekçisi. (2024, February 2). Disco Elysium and the meaningfulness of delusions. Medium. https://deluzyoner42.medium.com/disco-elysium-and-the-meaningfulness-of-delusions-acb8550f6440

Diggins, C. (2021, June 22). I don't want to get better – I want to get worse. Alittleperspective.substack.com. https://alittleperspective.substack.com/p/i-dont-want-to-get-better-i-want

Euro Brady. (n.d.). *Home* [YouTube channel]. YouTube. Retrieved May 2, 2025, from https://www.youtube.com/@eurobrady

Ferchaud, A., Seibert, J., Sellers, N., & Escobar Salazar, N. (2020). Reducing mental health stigma through identification with video game avatars with mental illness. Frontiers in Psychology, 11. https://doi.org/10.3389/fpsyg.2020.02240

GameSpot. "The feature that almost sank Disco Elysium | Audio Logs." *YouTube*, 12 Jan. 2020, www.youtube.com/watch?v=9X0-W5erEXw

Geography of Robots. (2022). *Norco* [PC]. Raw Fury.

Go, S. (2022, January 14). Disco Elysium took me some time to get into. Medium; Avoider.net. https://medium.com/avoider-net/disco-elysium-took-me-some-time-to-get-into-6fd22c98cbda

Hellblade: Senua's Sacrifice [PC]. (2017). Ninja Theory.

Izual. (2019, July 15). Choose your own misadventure – Part 1. DiscoElysium.com. https://discoelysium.com/devblog/2019/07/15/choose-your-own-misadventure-part-1

Izual. (2019, July 23). Choose your own misadventure – Part 2. DiscoElysium.com. https://discoelysium.com/devblog/2019/07/23/choose-your-own-misadventure-part-2

Jackson, G. (2019, December 13). Disco Elysium developers shout out Marx and Engels in Game Awards victory speech. Kotaku. https://kotaku.com/disco-elysium-developers-shout-out-marx-and-engels-1840403603

Jump Over the Age. (2022). *Citizen Sleeper* [PC]. Fellow Traveler.

Lisa: the painful [PC]. (2014). Dingaling Productions.

Klimczyk, P. (2021). The experience of playing video games as a possible building block for life story narratives. Polskie Forum Psychologiczne, 26(2). https://doi.org/10.34767/PFP.2021.02.05

Knox, R. (1929). Introduction. In R. Knox & H. Harrington (Eds.), The Best English Detective Stories of 1928. Horace Liveright.

Kuhn, B. (2022, August 8). Disco Elysium taught me how to live. Pro Game Guides. https://progameguides.com/disco-elysium/disco-elysium-taught-me-how-to-live/

Magestro, T. (2021, February 28). How Disco Elysium taught me it's okay to be broken. Start 2 Continue. https://start2continue.com/metzge/how-disco-elysium-helped-me-be-okay-with-being-broken/

Morton, L. (2019, November 6). Disco Elysium interview – I don't want to be this kind of animal anymore. VG247. https://www.vg247.com/disco-elysium-intrusive-thoughts

PENTIMENT [PC]. (2022). Obsidian Entertainment. Xbox Game Studios.

Rijnders, F. (2023). Meaning-making processes in successful commercial games: A Dark Souls and Disco Elysium case study. Utrecht University. https://studenttheses.uu.nl/bitstream/handle/20.500.12932/45145/Master%20Thesis%20-%20Frans%20Rijnders%20-%209354670.pdf

Spies, T. (2021). "Making sense in a senseless world": Disco Elysium's absurd hero. Baltic Screen Media Review, 9(1), 80–89. https://doi.org/10.2478/bsmr-2021-0008

Walker, I. (2021, April 6). When my Disco Elysium character gave up I was like yeah, I get it. Kotaku. https://kotaku.com/when-my-disco-elysium-character-gave-up-i-was-like-yeah-1846624407

Wiltshire, A. (2020, January 9). The making of Disco Elysium: How ZA/UM created one of the most original RPGs of the decade. GamesRadar+. https://www.gamesradar.com/the-making-of-disco-elysium-how-zaum-created-one-of-the-most-original-rpgs-of-the-decade/

Woodford, D. (2019, November 13). The political alignment system. ZA/UM. https://web.archive.org/web/20201201234721/https://zaumstudio.com/2019/11/13/the-political-alignment-system/

ZA/UM. (2018). DISCO ELYSIUM BOX ART [Electronic resource]. https://store.steampowered.com/news/app/632470/view/4740557883125835404

ZA/UM. (2021). DISCO ELYSIUM: THE FINAL CUT [PC].

# Appendix

# Contributors

**Accettulli, Samantha** is a therapist and owner of Conversation Tree Therapy in Austin, Texas. She specializes in working with neurodivergent clients, especially those with autism and ADHD, as well as clients working in creative fields. She brings her experience of working in the arts and her knowledge and understanding of the importance of media to her work with clients and believes that the entertainment we connect with and the lessons we learn about ourselves through it can promote greater understanding and healing.

**Alvarez Igarzábal, Federico** is Professor of Digital Media & Game Studies at the University of Fine Arts Essen (HBK Essen). His research explores the aesthetics of games and play, combining theoretical and experimental approaches. Over the past decade, he has focused on the temporal aesthetics of video games, analyzing the medium's temporal characteristics and how they interact with our perception of time. His book TIME AND SPACE IN VIDEO GAMES. A COGNITIVE-FORMALIST APPROACH was published by transcript in 2019. Federico was also involved in the EU-funded project VIRTUALTIMES, whose aim was to develop virtual environments to treat psychopathologies like depression through the manipulation of time perception. In his current research project, *The Playing Mind*, Federico investigates the mental state of play, aiming to provide a cognitive account of this multifaceted cultural phenomenon. Website: federicoalvarez.com

**Bonenfant, Maude** is Full Professor in the Department of Social and Public Communication at the Université du Québec à Montréal (UQAM) and has a doctorate in semiotics. She holds the Canada Research Chair in Games, Technologies and Society, co-directs the Research Laboratory in Social Media and Gamification, and directs the Homo Ludens research group on games and communication. Her research focuses on the study of games, the social dimensions of communication technologies, online communities, social networks, big data, and artificial intelligence.

**Bowman, Nicholas D.** (PhD, Michigan State University, USA) is Professor in the S.I. Newhouse School of Public Communications at Syracuse University, USA. His research is focused on the cognitive, emotional, physical, and social demands of interactive media such as video games and extended reality applications. He also studies nostalgia and entertainment media, as well as how gamers and XR users form sense of place in persistent online worlds and spaces. He is the former Fulbright Wu Jing-Jyi Arts and Culture Fellow in Taiwan and the most recent editor of JOURNAL OF MEDIA PSYCHOLOGY, and the launch editor of GLOBAL PERSPECTIVES IN COMMUNICATION.

**Comeau, Chad** is a researcher at the Cologne Game Lab (TH Köln, Germany), creative director at Reframe Games, and leads interactive cultural projects through his company Fring Frang Games. Bringing over a decade of professional experience in game design, project management and languages, Chad tackles various societal and cultural issues in his work. In the cultural sector, Chad has led many participatory projects in his hometown of Clare, Nova Scotia, including CLAREVOYANCE, an adventure video game made in collaboration with over 130 community members contributing performances, music, art, and stories; CLARE CUISINE +, a cross-cultural interactive cooking app highlighting local food and international dishes from newcomers; and À TCHI?, a fun and accessible cultural card game based on a local tradition funded by the local university and a successful Kickstarter campaign. In Europe, Chad graduated with a bachelor's degree in Digital Games with focus on Game Design from the Cologne Game Lab, where he now works as a researcher developing serious games. His experience includes ANTURA & THE LETTERS, a language-learning app, where he coordinated the award-winning version for Ukrainian refugees, adding 6 new languages in three months to respond to the Ukrainian crisis in 2022. He later served as coordinator and game designer on the ISEDA VICTIM INTERVIEW SIMULATOR, working with 15 partner institutions across Europe to develop innovative, victim-centred training software to promote better practices towards victims of domestic and gender-based violence. He is now a partner on the SOILSCAPE project, organizing events and supporting creators making games promoting soil literacy and awareness.

**Dunlap, Kelli** (PsyD, MA) is the executive director at Take This, the original mental health and games non-profit, and brings on over a decade of experience working at the intersection of mental health and games. In addition to her work at Take This, Dr. Dunlap is a licensed clinical psychologist, holds a Masters in game design, and serves as a researcher-in-residence at American University's Game Center. Her collaborations include NIMH, UNESCO, VOX Media, and U.S. Congressional staffers. Dr. Dunlap is an internationally recognized researcher and speaker on the intersection of games and mental health, especially pertaining to mental health representation in games and ethical game design.

**Genvo, Sébastien** is a professor at the University of Lorraine and affiliated with the Centre for Research on Mediation. A game designer at Ubisoft in 2001–2002, he defended the first thesis (2006) in France on video games. His work focuses on the artistic and cultural issues in the field, notably developing the concept of expressive games. In this context, he conducts research and creative activities that have led to the development of two independent games, KEYS OF A GAMESPACE (2011) and LIE IN MY HEART (2019). He is head of the Expressive Gamelab, a platform for video game analysis and creation.

**Guardiola, Emmanuel** is a veteran of the video game industry with more than 30 major titles published for publishers such as Ubisoft and independent studios. He has worked on licenses in various genres, including FAR CRY, PRINCE OF PERSIA, SPLINTER CELL, and FRANK HERBERT'S DUNE. At Ubisoft, after conducting research on video game design and emotions or meaning, he was one of the creators of the Game For Everyone brand, focused on how to bring concrete benefits to users. Emmanuel Guardiola holds a PhD in computer science and is now professor at the Cologne Game Lab, TH Köln (Cologne University of Applied Sciences, Germany). In the field of game design research, he is interested in models, processes, characteristics of the gameplay experience, and how we can apply these findings to education, health, psychology, or humanitarian causes. Regularly funded by national, European, and international grants, he has won more than 10 awards, such as the Game For Change Europe Award, the eVirtuos R&D Award, and the Interactive Author of the Year Award from the SACD (Society of Dramatic Authors and Composers). His ANTURA & THE LETTERS project, winner of the international EduApp4Syria call and an Erasmus+ grant, is aimed at refugee children and uses mobile games to promote Arabic literacy and psychosocial well-being. The game is currently being used in the field and has nearly 500,000 users. Antura has received many international awards in the field of education and humanitarian aid, including from the Red Cross and the UNHCR. His last project, the VICTIM INTERVIEW SIMULATOR, aims to train police officers to manage the psychological state of a survivor during initial contact. It was funded by an EU Horizon grant and is used by police authorities in several countries.

**Hodge, Sarah** (Ph.D., CPsychol, SFHEA) is a cyberpsychology researcher with a focus on gaming and gambling. Through exploring the interplay between human factors and game design in Human Computer Interaction (HCI) research, she has specifically explored game features (such as loot boxes), decision making and morality, transparency, and overlaps between gaming and gambling. She also conducts specific work on the player side of HCI research, exploring demographic factors, gaming experiences, digital addiction, engagement, moral development, and nostalgia. She utilises technology-driven methods to enhance our understanding of HCI by working with interdisciplinary teams of academics, industry partners, local businesses, game developers and designers, to create purpose-made games and Virtual Reality simulations for research and education. Such work and interdisciplinary teams have enabled her to explore how to psychologically support users, develop training and education, specifically focusing on the concepts of digital resilience in children and young people's technology use. Currently, she is an Academic Leader in the School of Sciences at Bath Spa University, United Kingdom. Email: s.hodge@bathspa.ac.uk

**Johann, Carmen** is a game designer, UX designer, and researcher in the field of digital learning, specializing in user-centered learning systems, serious games, and interactive educational media. After completing her studies and working internationally as a game and UX designer, she spent many years at the Cologne Game Lab, an institute at the Technical University of Cologne, where she worked in interdisciplinary teams as a lead game designer and project manager, and as a lecturer. As part of numerous nationally funded research projects, she led the design, implementation, and evaluation of digital learning and training systems. A particular focus was on Project SOLVE, an interdisciplinary federal project that dealt with the development and piloting of an innovative game-based prevention measure for young people at increased risk of substance abuse and addiction. As Game Design and UX Lead, she was responsible for all user research, the development of personas and user journeys, and the design of interactive prototypes and feedback systems. Her work contributed significantly to the development of learning-effective and motivating interaction concepts based on the principles of human-centered design. In addition, she researched and taught on topics such as serious game design, gamification, digital learning environments, and user experience in educational contexts. Alongside her academic work, as co-founder of the creative agency Pixelbeschleuniger, she led numerous projects in the fields of digital communication, user interface design, and interactive learning media. Her research is characterized by the combination of design practice, empirical user research, and theoretical reflection. The aim of her work is to develop digital learning environments that provide intuitive spaces for humans, which offer new worlds to explore and shape one's own being.

**Kelly, Danielle** (Dr.) (she/her) is a cyberpsychologist and Lecturer in Psychology at the University of the West of Scotland, UK. Dr. Kelly completed her Ph.D. in 2018 at the University of Stirling, exploring the individual and social complexities of metacognition in education-based learning. From there, Dr. Kelly's passion for gaming led to applying her experimental expertise to the area of cyberpsychology, specifically with a focus on cyberdeviance (e.g. cyber-stalking/cyberflashing behaviour) and perceptions of gender in gaming culture. Dr. Kelly's work has expanded to investigate the psychological factors that underpin gender stereotypes in gaming communities using experimental and qual-itative methods. Her work aims to improve an awareness of barriers to inclusion in the gaming domain, making gaming communities more accessible and safer for everyone.

**Kerttula, Tero** is postdoctoral researcher at the University of Jyväskylä, Finland. He has expertise in the fields of online streaming and media culture. His PhD dissertation in 2022 discussed video game-related YouTube videos and online streams as a part of current video game culture. Kerttula has also studied and lectured about media history of video games, media journalism, media literacy and competitive gaming. He has also published numerous articles, book chapters, and educational work about the said themes. Along with his academic work, Kerttula has also worked for two decades as a freelance journalist for different video game publications as well. Currently he is working on different themes regarding the history of video game journalism and video games portraying more difficult themes of human life.

**King, Jordan** is a PhD candidate in the School of Psychology at Bournemouth University, UK. His doctoral research explores the triggers of nostalgia in video games, using a mixed-methods approach to examine the affective responses players have toward their bygone digital worlds. He has shared this work widely through public engagement, including interactive demonstrations, oral presentations, and sessions with undergraduate psychology students. Jordan is a member of the BPS Cyberpsychology Section and has served as a reviewer for the student journal PRESS START, which publishes research on video games. His interest in video game psychology began during his BSc studies at Bournemouth University, particularly through coursework on the psychology of social media and video games unit. Email: jking1@bournemouth.ac.uk

**Leech, Christopher** (PhD) is a Lecturer of Psychology at the University of Brighton. Chris' PhD is in psychology looking at video games and student mental health. Chris is a person with Albinism, which means he's visually impaired/legally blind. Chris is a content creator, podcast host, author, presenter, and accessibility consultant. Chris combines elements of mental health awareness, research, and accessibility throughout all his content. Chris is also avidly involved with various organisations, including Take This, Safe in Our World, Impact, Many Cats Studios, and Limit Break (as part of the Accessibility committee).

**Lhotellier, Clara** is a master's student in Communications at Université du Québec à Montréal (UQAM), specializing in video games and gamification. She was research assistant for the Canada Research Chair in Games, Technologies and Society and now works as a junior user researcher at Eidos-Montréal.

**Rüth, Marco** is a postdoctoral researcher and lecturer at the University of Cologne with a focus on media psychology, educational technology, and digital games. He received his doctorate in psychology for his work on theoretical progress and educational practice regarding learning and teaching with digital games. He has coordinated several projects on the design, development, and evaluation of digital learning tools in teacher education, medical education, and interdisciplinary settings. With his interdisciplinary background in psychology, cognitive science, and neural and behavioral sciences, he aims to investigate and advance the potential of digital and game-based interventions. Website: https://linktr.ee/marcorueth

**Schütt, Kerstin.** With Bachelor's degrees in computer science and game design, Kerstin took the leap into freelancing in 2017, working on a range of projects before focusing on DURU, a colorful serious game about depression. In 2020, together with two fellow graduates, she co-founded the indie game studio Twisted Ramble Games. Their debut title, DURU, was released in 2023 and has since been nominated for and honored with multiple awards. Although her co-founders have since pursued different career paths, Kerstin continues to forge her own way in the games industry under her new label Infinite Retries. Her passion lies at the intersection of creativity, mental health awareness, and interactive storytelling. She is especially dedicated to exploring how games can both entertain and spark meaningful conversations about complex topics. Beyond development, Kerstin is committed to education and knowledge-sharing. She teaches courses and leads workshops for students at various levels, from high school to university, and views teaching as an extension of her creative practice. Whether in the classroom or through her projects, she aims to inspire others to experiment, reflect, and use games as a tool for both self-expression and social impact.

**Simond, Stefan Heinrich** (PhD) is an academic lecturer in the game design program at IU (International University of Applied Sciences). He completed his doctorate degree, titled PIXELATED MADNESS. THE CONSTRUCTION OF MENTAL ILLNESSES AND PSYCHIATRIC INSTITUTIONS IN VIDEO GAMES with summa cum laude. His current research focuses on video games as spaces of resonance and the construction of martial arts in video games.

**Srirachanikorn, Richy** is a PhD candidate in the Social and Cultural Analysis program at Concordia University, Montreal. He studies how online groups and grassroots communities build towards a collective future, using their nostalgia for the past "the way it could have been". In 2022, Richy co-founded the Nostagain Network, North America's first student-led research collective studying the generative potentials of nostalgia. Besides nostalgia and video games, Richy studies time as a method of social control, Hikikomori and digital technologies, and games as an object of the past.

**Thomas, Bethany** (she/her) is a postgraduate researcher (PhD) at Edge Hill University, UK, and assistant lecturer at Arden University. Throughout her studies, Beth has focused on gender identity in stigmatised settings, with a particular focus on stereotypes and identity. This is reflected in her current research as part of her doctoral studies, which explore the intersection between gender identity and gamer identity, investigating the efficacy of various theoretical frameworks from social psychology as processes involved in the construction of gamer identity, in order to establish the theoretical basis from which female gamers may be better understood. Beth's work combines underpinnings from social, cyber and feminist psychology drawing from predominantly reflexive qualitative research methods. Beth is also an ambassador for Women in Games (WIGJ), and member of the BPS Cyberpsychology Committee.

**Tillmanns, Katharina** is a researcher, designer, and curator working at the intersection of games, psychology, and embodied media. She is a lecturer at the Cologne Game Lab, TH Köln, and a doctoral candidate at University of Cologne where her research explores Mixed Reality design with a focus on affect, emotional engagement, and user well-being. Tillmanns' academic work is grounded in creative production and cultural mediation. As co-founder and co-curator of Games for Change Europe, she established a platform for dialogue on how games can serve as cultural artifacts and catalysts for social change. Her own projects span a wide range of formats, from historical location-based AR games such as HisToGo and Border Zone—which combine walking, role-play, and situated storytelling to support affective, body-based learning—to collaborative VR performances and experimental simulators that explore synesthetic and somatic dimensions of play. In addition to her research and design work, she has contributed to the international games culture as a festival director and curator, notably through the Notgames Fest trilogy (2011–2015) and the more recent SomaFest, a platform dedicated to somatics and immersive media. Across her projects and publications, Tillmanns advances the idea of games as both artistic and epistemic media, with the potential to support psychological insight, foster empathy, and open new pathways for education and well-being.

**Vial, Élisa** is a PhD candidate in semiotic studies at the Université du Québec à Montréal (UQAM). She studies representation of the psychiatric asylum and hospitals in video games. She is a member of the Homo Ludens research group on games and communication and a research assistant for the Canada Research Chair in Games, Technologies and Society.

**Wulf, Tim** (Ph.D., University of Cologne, Germany) is a researcher at the intersection of media studies, communication science, and psychology. His research interests include media-induced nostalgia, the uses and effects of video games, and persuasion through narrative media and storytelling. After his PhD at the University of Cologne in Germany in 2018, Tim Wulf held a PostDoc position at the Department of Media and Communication at the Ludwig-Maximilians-University in Munich, Germany. In 2021, he was granted the Kyoon Hur Dissertation Award of the Mass Communication Division of the International Communication Association for his research on media-induced nostalgia. Currently, he is working as a Senior Advertising Researcher at RTL Data (RTL Deutschland GmbH). Website: https://www.tim-wulf.de. Email: wulf.tim@gmail.com